It's OK To Eat

Be fit, healthy, and NOT on a diet

By

Annette Mucci-Haggerty

© 2002 by Annette Mucci-Haggerty.
All rights reserved.

No part of this book may be reproduced, stored in a retrieval system, or transmitted by any means, electronic, mechanical, photocopying, recording, or otherwise, without written permission from the author.

ISBN: 1-4033-1293-1

This book is printed on acid free paper.

1stBooks - rev. 04/19/02

Acknowledgments

First - I would like to thank Sherry and Auntie Marcy, the two people who have always believed in me and supported me in all of my wacky ideas and plans.

Second - I would like to thank my husband, Danny for putting up with all of my latest wacky ideas and plans.

Third - I would like to thank Donna Toto for her help with editing and James Fitzgerald for his help with the cover design. Also, thank you to Paula for helping me with my website.

Introduction

Let's rewind back to about 1980ish. I was 19 years old and driving home alone after dropping off my clubbing buddy. We'll call her Darlene. She was about 5' 5', petite blonde and a man magnet. I am 5' ½", weighed about 150 pounds at the time and attracted very few men. Ever. You could say I was a Big Mac magnet.

Just that evening I had picked Darlene up and we went to a local dive to hook up with an old friend of my big brother. The kids called him "Fleabag". He was gorgeous.

Fleabag had actually been calling me on the phone asking where I was going and what I was doing for the last couple of weeks. Could it be that he was actually interested in me? I had begged Darlene to come out to the specified place so I could meet up with this cute guy.

Of course, she said yes. I had dressed up in my favorite red disco dress with spaghetti straps and plunging neckline to show off my then "B" sized breasts. (Believe it or not, B was the biggest I ever got and that was only thanks to the chubbiness. I hadn't had any children then, so they were still kind of perky). She wore whatever. What difference did it make? She always looked good.

We arrived at the bar. I was so freaked that a friend of my big brother finally noticed me and wanted to meet me. Maybe now that I was older he no longer saw me as a kid? I was very nervous and excited. After all, I had been watching this guy ignore me for over three years. As it turns out, I would watch him ignore me yet again.

You guessed it. It wasn't me that he wanted to hook up with... It was Darlene.

I tried to hide my disappointment by sucking down a few Black Russians. I even tried to get a good flirt session going with another cute guy. Hey, maybe I could make Fleabag jealous. When I realized that the guy I had been talking to had never once looked at my face, only the spot where my breasts were being held in place by my red spandex dress, I hit bottom.

There was nothing and no one (certainly not myself) there to break my fall.

I told the happy couple that I wanted to leave. Of course, Fleabag didn't have a ride so I was obliged to drive the two of them home. They both ended up sitting in the front seat with me. After all, Fleabag couldn't possibly sit in the back of my 1968 piece of crap Rambler station wagon all by himself! I did, however, draw the line at chauffeuring the two of them home while they made out in the back seat. I wasn't a complete fool.

Try driving home after about 5 Black Russians (I could really put it away then), tears in your eyes the whole time, with your good friend and the guy who you had left your house expecting to be with that evening (need I remind you about the 3 year crush?) flirting in the front seat like you didn't even exist.

It was a blast.

Needless to say, I spent the entire ride wishing God would come and take me right then and there. Even then, I was not the type to have bad wishes towards them. After all, it wasn't their fault I was a fat slob. I couldn't blame him for using me to get at adorable Darlene, could I? (To give her a little bit of credit - she didn't end up going out with him again. Although I wonder why she went out with him at all?)

After I dropped them both off, I drove home just praying to God to give me the courage to fall asleep at the wheel and maybe ram a tree or something. I didn't want any innocents on the street to die, but had decided that was unlikely since there was almost no traffic at 2am. I was so tired anyway. It would be easy to just drop off to sleep. So easy. Of course, no one would miss me - especially not Fleabag.

That was rock bottom. I will never forget that experience.

God did not grant me my wish. Instead, I ended up doing the bravest thing of all. I made it home in one piece and continued to live.

Now here I am, 20 years later. I'm married for the second time. My first husband and I are great friends and are raising our two wonderful (I swear) children together and doing a hell of a job - with the help of my new husband, my ex's girlfriend, and some family members.

I couldn't tell you what I weigh. I threw the scale out a long time ago. But I'm a size 6. And get this: I'm an aerobics instructor!!!

But the most important part of this story is that I truly love myself. I get a real kick out of ME. Believe it or not, I am not on a diet nor have I been since a short while after my second child was born.

As the mother of one of my childhood friends used to say, "Put that in your pipe and smoke it."

1

Why Diets Don't Work

My story

I still remember vividly the day I first realized that I was fat. It was the beginning of the summer after sixth grade. I had been very active up until fifth grade, doing gymnastics on the lawn every chance I could get. During that winter, however, I had dislocated my elbow during a Saturday open gym at the High School. That put me in a cast and slowed me down for quite a while.

I had never in my life worried about weight and had no idea about how metabolism works. I had no idea that if you sat still (or went through puberty, for heaven's sake) things would start to change. Well, change they did.

I will never forget the beautiful bikini that I had carelessly worn the summer before the accident. It was made of a striking rainbow floral fabric and it looked so good on me. I felt a bit sexy for the first time in my life. Well, after sixth grade was over I eagerly dug my gorgeous bikini out of the drawer - and cried when I saw how I looked in it.

There I was, standing in my mother's room looking at myself in the big mirror. I had bulges around the edges of the elastic on the hips and legs of the bikini bottom. I had not been prepared for this. I had always been a skinny kid and naively had no notion of how a person could gain weight.

For the first time in my life (but sure as heck not the last) I was ashamed of my body. It was awful.

My fate as a "chub" (or so I believed) was sealed when a boy at a 7th grade party dubbed me "The Elephant in High Heels". (I had borrowed those shoes from my sister, thinking that they made me look more mature - and thinner since I was taller with them on. Apparently, I was mistaken.

So began years of having an eating problem and as many years (somewhere around 18 years total, I'm thinking) of dieting. I spent every waking moment at some stage of a diet. At any given time I was starting a diet, quitting a diet, restarting a diet, or cheating on a diet. I counted calories, fat grams, carbohydrates and glasses of water. You name it - I tried it.

I seesawed with weight all through high school and after. I had at least three different sizes of jeans in my drawer at all times. I blamed everything on my heaviness. I know that I had an attractive face and I did manage to get my small share of boyfriends but still I always blamed my fat ass and thighs when things didn't work out.

It wasn't until much later in life that I realized that being skinny does not a happy person make.

My Theories

Let's suppose that I decide to go on a diet. I want you to think about the usual reasons one would chose to go on a diet. Probably because I think I'm overweight, out of shape, not healthy. The bottom line is that food has become much too important in my life. I'm spending too much of my valuable time thinking about food. Most likely I've been using food to fulfill some need that I have - which is probably NOT the need to fuel my body.

Annette Mucci-Haggerty

When I agree to go on a diet, I am continuing to make food too much of an issue. Now I'm going to spend even more time thinking about food. I am constantly asking myself (probably others too) questions such as: What can I eat? What can't I eat? What did I eat so far? *Why* did I eat that? *And damn it, when can I eat again?*

Already, something is wrong. Maybe I'm crazy, but is our goal to spend the rest of our lives calculating day by day the amount of food we ate, the calories, the fat grams so that we can be comfortable in our bodies? Doesn't that sound like a life sentence in some strange prison?

Or is the goal to get to the point where food doesn't matter? That wonderful place where we only think about food because our stomachs are saying, "Hello! I need fuel or I'm going to crash. I don't care what it is, as long as it fills me up and gives me some vitamins. Thank you very much." Then we can spend our precious time taking care of important things like being the best we can be - doing our jobs, taking care of our families, feeling **good.** Oh yes, feeling **GOOD**!

Do you have to constantly monitor every breath that you take? Doesn't your body take care of that all by itself? Well, I'm proposing that your body is completely capable of taking care of the food intake as well - but only if you allow it to. We have been conditioned from the time we were young that we have to keep track of what we eat and how much and how often. I say no to this. I say (and have proven this in my own life) that we only need to let nature take its course, listen to our bodies and its needs and we will be A-OK.

Now let's review what the results of trying to diet can sometimes be.

We can invent an average person. We'll name her Betty. She is a wonderful mother of three children and she works part time at the school to make extra money and be near her kids. She's awesome.

The only problem, according to her, is that she is about 30 pounds overweight. She hates to look at herself and hates even more getting dressed in the morning because she never knows what's going to fit, never mind what might be comfortable. Her husband loves her but can't help but make little comments about how good she used to look in high school, before she married him and got pregnant. *Thank you, honey. You are so sweet.*

Anyway, Betty is starting a diet for maybe the hundredth time in the past ten years. She chose to limit her calories to 1200 a day and try to keep her fat grams to 15. Good for her, you say.

Well, her day starts out wonderfully. She has a bowl of Special K (she likes the commercials) with skim milk. She wanted to put a banana in it, but has been told somewhere along the line that bananas have a lot of sugar. No problem, it wasn't all that bad plain.

That gets her to about 8:30am. She's at the school now and doing her usual great job but now she's starting to get hungry. Too bad for her. She'll just have to suck it up until 10:00 am when she can have her snack - one (1) delicious apple.

It's OK to Eat
Be Fit, Healthy, and NOT on a Diet

Well, stomach growling, our Betty makes it until the designated time. *This timing and planning is kind of fun,* she thinks, *like a game.* Boy, that apple was looking good and tasting good. But unfortunately, it just didn't do the job.

Our Betty is still starving.

Now there is another unfortunate part to this story. Poor Betty is having quite the inner conversation with herself. It goes something like this:

*Oh my God. I'm so hungry. I've done so good this far and I don't want to blow it. I can't stand my clothes, I can't stand my body, I can't stand **myself!** I have to be good. But boy, would I love a Hershey bar. Or maybe just a nice bag of Fritos… no, no, NO!*

No more Hershey bars for me. I'm going to be a good girl and be hungry for a while. It won't kill me and I'm sure I'll get used to it. Just wait until I get on that scale and find out that I've lost a pound, or even a half-pound! Then it will get easier.

That little pep talk works until lunch. Good for her. Lunch consists of a tuna fish sandwich (low-fat mayo, duh) on whole wheat bread and a diet coke. Very good so far.

Now it's 3:15PM. School is over and she's on her way home with the kids. Things are beginning to get worse.

Chocolate cake would just be wonderful. Maybe if I could just have a bite or two, I would be fine. Then I could get my mind off of this whole thing and behave for the rest of the day. The kids would probably love it too.

She goes home and makes the cake. The kids are thrilled. They can't wait to get their hands on that thing. Betty is thinking that this was a great idea. Keeping herself busy baking the cake kept her from touching the bag of Fritos in the cabinet. Maybe she can just wait for her afternoon snack of Wheat Thins and forget about the cake. Yeah, that's it. Just give it to the kids.

Now it's 4:00pm. The cake is ready. The Wheat Thins did nothing to lessen her craving. The inner struggle continues:

*It's OK to Eat
Be Fit, Healthy, and NOT on a Diet*

I'm a fat pig. I don't need cake. I'll wait till dinner. It will be much more satisfying to fit into a size 6 than to eat a flipping piece of cake. I won't eat it.

End of story? No way!

Well, maybe just a bite or two. That will do the trick.

So, our friend serves her kids some cake and cuts just the tiniest sliver for herself. She even makes a cup of coffee to go with it. This is great.

Now the trouble really starts. That little voice inside begins to get mean. Or should I say, **meaner?**

*Oh-ho. Now you've done it. Ruined the **entire day!** Knew you couldn't do it. You couldn't keep your greedy little mouth off chocolate for one lousy day! Why even bother? You **are always going to be fat**! You're husband will probably leave you for some young, gorgeous, **skinny** thing. You are worthless. **Just admit it!***

Of course, the tape plays inside her head for much longer than that. She thinks: *Yup, today is gone. I might as well just forget it for today and eat even less tomorrow to make up for it. I am just a worthless fat slob. Might as well eat the rest of the cake since I'm going to starve tomorrow anyway. Besides, this whole thing is impossible anyway. I should just give up and accept the fact that I am fat.* ***I am always going to be fat.***

And that's just what she does. She eats a whole bunch of cake. Then she moves onto the Fritos. After dinner, she just has to have some ice cream for dessert. She can't just sit there and watch her husband and kids eat it. Tomorrow is another day.

You may think that I'm making fun of poor Betty. I am not. I have lived this scenario over and over again in my life. I ate an entire pizza one afternoon. I used to sit and stare at a doughnut, or some fries my stomach so full it **hurt,** and still I could not help but give in and eat the next thing that came along, whatever it was.

I used to wear pants that were so tight (I had made up my mind that I would NEVER buy a size 15 so I kept with the 13s even though they were too small) that I had to put them on damp so they would stretch out as they dried. This was really terrible in the summer time when it was humid. Try pulling on a damp pair of pants that are a size too small for you when it is about 90 degrees out. Not fun.

Now, back to why diets don't work.

Let us invent another nice person. Her name can be Joan. Joan has actually managed to stick to a diet for 6 months. She's looking awesome! She went from a size 13 down to a 5! No kidding! She went to bed hungry many a night but man, was it all worth it! She has arrived.

People are constantly telling her how wonderful she looks. She loves to go shopping and buy new clothes. Sexy jeans. She looks at her old clothes and can't believe that she ever was that huge.

She's still spending every day counting those calories, watching those fat grams. Can't take a chance on gaining anything back. She'll just have to accept the fact that she will never be able to have another piece of cheesecake again. Sorry - but it's much more fun being thin than eating cheesecake.

What's wrong with this picture? I'll tell you what's wrong.

Here is Joan, supposedly happy. And why shouldn't she be? She's thin! She did it! But wait a minute here!

She's still spending every waking minute of every day thinking about food.

Only now instead of thinking about what she ate and how fat she is, she's thinking about what she didn't eat and how great she's doing and basically stressing herself to death with worry about getting fat again!

Here's a snippet of her average conversation with a co-worker. "I'm so proud of myself. All I've eaten so far today is one waffle with sugarless syrup of course, and a half of a sandwich! Ok, I allowed myself two potato chips, but that's not bad, is it?" (Meanwhile, the co-worker can't get away from her fast enough. Who wants to hear someone's daily intake as a topic of conversation?)

Is this happiness? I DON'T THINK SO!

It's OK to Eat
Be Fit, Healthy, and NOT on a Diet

As far as I'm concerned these two people are both in the same boat. Granted, one is eating a lot, and one is hardly eating at all. What they have in common is that they are both concentrating totally on food. Are they free? NO WAY!

I'd bet my house that Joan is going to start putting on weight again within a couple of months. How do I know this? I've lived Joan's scenario also. I've been about 160 pounds and a size I-don't-want-to-talk-about-it and I've been 103 pounds and a size 3. (I think the size 3 lasted about a week). But no matter what size I was and what stage I was at, I was always thinking about food. Rarely did I eat simply because I was hungry. And worse, *never* did I stop eating because I was full.

My meals were ruled by RULES, guilt and self-abuse.

Now here is an interesting point that I observed over my years of eating and not eating which may help to explain another of the reasons that diets don't work:

Annette Mucci-Haggerty

Your body does not need or desire the same amount of food every day.

I saw this in action while married to my first husband. He was an athlete his whole life. He still plays basketball for fun and he has never been fat. Ever. He also installs carpets for a living, which is a physical job.

I would watch his eating habits and I noticed that some days he just would not stop eating. He would go literally from one meal to the next. He, of course, never worried about this. He was hungry and that was that.

On other days, he would not even eat two full meals. I would ask him if he was sick. "Nope," he would say. "I'm just not hungry today."

This was interesting. How come he didn't have to count calories and eat the same amount every day? This is when I began to realize that our bodies do a very good job of taking care of themselves if we allow them to.

It's OK to Eat
Be Fit, Healthy, and NOT on a Diet

Some days you may work off more calories due to exercise, stress, whatever, so maybe you need to eat more. On another, you may be relaxing by the pool (don't you wish) and food is not as necessary. Then there are those hormone days when I myself just can't get enough to eat for whatever reason.

The point is this: I don't believe that we were designed to eat the same measure of calories and fat grams, etc. every day. These needs change daily and it is just cruel and unusual punishment to try to stick to some diet that only allows you to eat the same small amount all of the time.

I'll never forget the last time that I went to one of those diet centers - you know the ones that sell you *their* food to eat - and I didn't lose any weight at all that week. I had confessed to my counselor that the only way I was able to stick to this starvation diet that she had me on was to promise myself that I would go eat a meal at McDonald's right after my weigh in. She told me that the McDonald's run was probably the reason that I hadn't lost even a half-pound in one whole week! Keep in mind that at this time I was working out for one hour every day and sticking to the diet every single day (I believe I was only allowed 1200 calories a day. Starvation.) and going to bed hungry every night. How could that one McDonald's run be hurting me?

Later in life, after I had learned more about metabolism, I realized that the reason I was not losing weight was because I was not eating ***enough.***

No wonder I couldn't stick with the diet center.

2

A Couple Of Ideas That It is Time To Let Go Of

My Story

I was 20 years old. I had just moved out of my parents house and into an apartment with a roommate. I felt like a grown up for the first time. When I first moved into this apartment, I had just lost some weight and was down to about a size 9, which for me was awesome.

I ran into this guy. His name was Peter. I hadn't seen him for a couple of years. He used to hang around outside my parents ice cream shop and talk to me. He was nice but he was a few years older and had not been interested in me (chubby as I was) when I had been in high school.

This guy Peter began showing up again while I was working. If it wasn't busy he would stick around and talk, just like he used to do. I told him about my new apartment, trying to impress him with how grown up I was. After he had come by quite a few times and I had dropped a few hints without being shot down, I got up the nerve to invite him over for dinner. He surprised me by accepting.

I had never cooked dinner for a man before and was completely excited about the whole thing. This was HUGE! Here was an older guy who had never been interested in me and he was coming to my apartment to have dinner with ME! Maybe all of that dieting had paid off.

I planned the meal for days. I spent a fortune on that meal. I baked a cheesecake from scratch the day before and almost killed my roommate when she had taken a strawberry off of the top and ruined the appearance. (What was wrong with her, anyway?) I made lasagna from home made spaghetti sauce, a huge bowl of meatballs and a salad. Then, of course, there was the cheesecake (I had managed to move the strawberries around and make it look presentable).

Then he knocked on my door. I was so nervous I could barely breath.

It's OK to Eat
Be Fit, Healthy, and NOT on a Diet

I showed him all of the food that I had painstakingly laid out on the table for him. He wasn't hungry yet, he said. Allrighty. I opened a bottle and we drank some wine.

After an hour or so, I asked him if he was ready to eat. Well actually, he told me, he wasn't hungry at all since he had been doing cocaine before he had gotten there. He proceeded to pull the little white envelope out of his pocket and asked me if I wanted any.

I was crushed about the food but shrugged it off. Well, I told myself, at least he was there - with me. We ended up drinking wine and doing a couple of lines until about 11pm.

That was when he began to kiss me all the while trying to get his hand inside my shirt. I told him "no thank you". I didn't want to do that. I didn't mind kissing though, so I let him keep kissing me. But he wouldn't stop trying to grab at my private places.

Apparently he hadn't come over to eat dinner. Apparently he had come over to party and get laid.

After about an hour of fending him off, I finally persuaded him to leave, although not in the way I should have. I should have booted his ass out the door and told him what a scumbag he was. But I wanted him to like me and to maybe come back (pathetic, I know) so I got rid of him nicely.

I spent over a week hoping and praying that he would come by the ice-cream shop or call me. Maybe he had come over to get laid but maybe he really liked me also? Wrong answer! He did not call, or ever again come by for an ice cream.

It only took me a few days to eat all of the lasagna.

And the meatballs.

And of course, the cheesecake.

My Theories

Here are a couple of things that I would advise you to get out of your head immediately, if not sooner.

1) I'm going to look better in… a few days, a week, or a month.

I call this thinking "Overnight Thinking".

I know you can't stand it another minute. The way you look. The way your clothes fit. How you feel about yourself. But (I know you don't want to hear this) you didn't get this way (I'm referring to whatever *way* you may be that you can't abide any longer) overnight. It took years of abuse, trying to diet, punishing yourself, trying to *be something* that you have decided - or have been told - that you are not, for you to get out of control. You cannot change everything in one day, one week, one month or maybe not even one year.

Now don't stop reading this book and throw it across the room in aggravation.

Giving up this Overnight Thinking will help you to succeed. It's the Overnight Thinking that got you backed up in the first place.

Think about it.

You decide that you can't stand yourself a moment longer. You put yourself on a ridiculously low calorie diet and maybe you even decide that are going to work out for an hour every day. By the end of the week, maybe you can lose five pounds. The more the better.

Don't you see that by setting yourself up with these unhealthy, unattainable goals that you are setting yourself up to be disappointed? All right, maybe you will stick to your starvation diet for the week, and even do the workouts. Maybe you will lose those five pounds or even more. Unfortunately however, you won't look like Julia Roberts in a week. You probably won't look like Julia Roberts in five years. Or like your best friend, the man magnet either.

You are not those people. ***You are your own special self.***

I'm sure you have already experienced what happens when you limit yourself so much that finally you can't stand it anymore. You go on a binge and eat everything in sight. Or when you've told yourself that you have to exercise for at least an hour and the thought so overwhelms you that you don't do anything at all. These are examples of what comes about when you expect to change your body overnight.

Remember all of the times you have tried to rush things only to end up getting frustrated and giving up? You checked the scale, the mirror, the clothes you were trying to fit into and it just didn't happen fast enough. So in the end, you decided you were fighting a losing battle and you quit.

Until you couldn't stand it anymore and you started all over again.

Why not accept a few new ideas - swallow them whole and start with an entirely different attitude? Why not praise yourself for every small victory, no matter what it is?

Why not try to take a whole bunch of successful small steps instead of one impossible giant leap?

There are two concepts that I'm trying to sell to you here. The first is to accept your own body's limitations. If you are short, you will not ever look like a model. If you are big breasted, you will never look like a ballet dancer. You want to learn to see your body in its best light. And remember, it really doesn't matter what you like or don't like about your shape. There are people out there who are attracted to all different things. Some men love big breasts. Others can't stand them. Some men only go for petite or short women.

Some men don't even look at skinny women. *Can you imagine that?*

The second concept is that no matter how far you have to go, the Overnight Thinking will only hurt you more than it will help. The desperate feeling that you can change (and all of those commercials promising huge weight loss in a week or less don't help any) overnight will only lead you to ultimate defeat. Not to mention the damage done to your insides by the starvation or the over-working out involved.

No one can climb a mountain by taking a huge jump. She can only do it one step at a time.

I have had to accept the fact that no matter how much I work out, no matter what size I may be I have thighs that would look one hell of a lot better on a tall person. They are in shape, muscular thighs but they don't belong on someone five feet one half inch tall. Oh well! Guess what? I have learned to appreciate my short thighs and apparently there are some men out there who seem to admire them too (my husband being one of them). Whatever. They are mine and no one else's and I'm going to keep them. Even if I could give them up, I'm going to keep them.

I will mention as a sidebar here that I have had some surgery done on my rear and thigh area. I want to be completely honest with you so that you will know that you can believe what I say.

What happened is this. Since I was up and down with weight from about age 12 until age 32 (including 2 pregnancies during which I gained at least 60 pounds), my skin lost its elasticity. To put it bluntly, my bum sagged down almost to my knees. No kidding. It was a nasty sight to behold. I decided that since I had never had the chance in my entire life to feel good in a pair of shorts or a bathing suit (remember the floral bikini?) that I would go have that extra skin removed. It is called a buttocks lift.

So I visited my friendly plastic surgeon and she very nicely cut a line from one hip to the other in the back and removed the extra 8 inches of skin. She also insisted that she would do a bit of lipo-suction to even everything off. Who was I to say no?? What I'm left with is a scar the travels in a large V-shape from one side of my hips to the other. In my eyes this very large scar is still much smaller that the one I had from all of my seesawing weight battles. That particular scar went from my waist all the way down to my knees!

I am not sorry that I did this but I want to point out that she still couldn't give me the tiny little ballerina thighs that I had always wanted. Nor would I have had her do such a thing. I just wanted her to make me look the way I would have looked if I had never had an eating problem in the first place.

I wanted to tell you about this so that it wouldn't come out some other time in the future and make me look like some sort of cheater. The bottom line is this: I no longer spend any of my time thinking about food. It does not run my life, except to be a need that I have to take care of or I will die from starvation.

Enough about my saggy rear end. Here is another thing that I think you must do.

2) *Throw your scale into the trash.*

It's OK to Eat
Be Fit, Healthy, and NOT on a Diet

Counting pounds will only cause you aggravation and frustration. Think about it. How many times have you dutifully counted your calories, walked your 45 minutes, drank your eight glasses of water all the while looking forward to the next morning when you can wake up and get the good news. Maybe you lost a half-pound, or maybe even an entire pound in one day!

What you actually find out is that you didn't lose anything at all. Maybe that little needle even moved just the tiniest bit the *other way*! You want to scream. You want to cry. You did all of the little tricks that you know are supposed to help. You emptied your bladder before getting on the scale - stripped yourself of every single piece of clothing. You even let out your breath before the big weigh-in. Still you didn't lose even an ounce.

What feelings now rise to the surface? Feelings of failure? Thoughts like: *maybe I'll just chuck the whole diet in the trash and eat an entire pizza for lunch?* (Been there. Done that). Or worse, *I'll just eat nothing today. I'll make sure that needle will move tomorrow.*

Or how about another scenario? You did manage to lose a pound in one day. Now you probably think you have to eat even less today to insure that you don't gain it back - even though you are hungry as hell.

Well, my friends. I say get rid of the scale. Who cares how much you weigh? All that truly matters is that you look and feel wonderful. Right? I've always said, I wouldn't care if I weighed three hundred pounds if I could fit into a size 5.

Let's not forget one really important fact here. Muscle weighs three times more than fat. So if you are working out in any way at all, you could actually be gaining weight while you are getting smaller. No lie. I weigh about 7 pounds more now that I would have in the past even though I wear about the same size (except now I'm in misses sizes instead of juniors - gotta love that). I know lots of people who can tell you the same thing. Ask your friends who go to the gym.

The scale only promotes the thinking that we are trying to get rid of. That good old Overnight Thinking.

You will not succeed in getting out of the diet rut forever if you don't stop looking for immediate results.

Again, I know that this concept is probably the hardest one for you to swallow but try to look at it this way: You have been using the "as soon as possible" idea for so long and where has it gotten you? How much time has gone by and you are still in the same boat? And if you have lost some weight, aren't you tired of thinking about it and worrying about it all of the time?

Don't you want a break, for heaven's sake?

3) *Try to put a stop to the "Woe is me" thinking.*

You may not be one of those people who walks around feeling sorry for yourself all of the time. If you are not, then you go girl! I do know that it is extremely difficult if you are overweight and not liking yourself all that much to *not* feel sorry for yourself.

There is nothing wrong with feeling sad. Quite a bit of our troubles come from doing things to *keep* from feeling sad - eating, drinking, spending, etc. when we should just sit still and feel sad and get it over with. However, continuously wallowing in self-pity will not solve your problem. Your goal here is to feel good about yourself, which will hopefully result in the confidence in yourself and your body to take care of your needs, which will then result in giving yourself a break.

Wallowing does NOT make one feel good about oneself. I will go out on a limb here and point out that self-pity probably contributes to quite a few of those pigging out episodes, does it not?

Instead of complaining about your situation, why not just focus on your future? Why not remind yourself of your good qualities, your unlimited potential and your desire to be the best that you can be, or the fact that you already are pretty damn good? Focus on what you can do to change your attitude RIGHT NOW, instead of wasting time feeling sorry for yourself.

Take a walk.

It's OK to Eat
Be Fit, Healthy, and NOT on a Diet

3

New Ideas to Replace Those Old Ones

My Story

I lasted in that apartment where I had my big night with the lovely Peter for about three months. I dated some men - invited a few of them over, but nothing worked out for me. Maybe I had watched too many of those movies where the girls just jump into bed with the guy at the beginning and all goes well from there. I don't think that I actually had sex with any of my men, but I think that they wanted me to and so I ended up feeling bad that I had somehow led them on and then worse when they never called me again even though I was a "good girl". I guess you could say that I was torn between my desire to be a sexy, attractive "woman" and my desire to be what I thought a "good girl" should be. During that three-month period I gained at least 25 pounds back. Needless to say, I was miserable.

The fall of that same year, I did the smartest thing I had ever done up to that point. I moved far away to Colorado. Luckily for me, my sister had been transferred there and so I was able to move in with her until I could manage on my own. That move was the beginning of the end of my weight problem and my eating problem (don't forget, these are two separate issues). Getting away from my parents and all of the people whom I felt had stuck me in the "chubby and not popular" category helped immensely. Of course, I didn't realize how much I had contributed to being stuck. I had needed a new beginning and there it was.

Out in Colorado I was able to see myself in a new light. I made friendships with people who judged me not on my weight, or how they had known me previously. They did not know my past and so accepted me on my own terms.

And they liked me!

Keep in mind I still was nowhere near thin at this point. In fact, I was at one of my chubbiest times of my life, with the exception of when I was pregnant years later. Could it be that I was likeable and attractive even though I was chubby!

It's OK to Eat
Be Fit, Healthy, and NOT on a Diet

I met new men and they called me when they said they would. They took me out on dates. I actually turned some of them down, since I just wasn't attracted or knew that they weren't for me. This was a new experience for me. Logically, I realized that there was no difference between the new men I met in Denver and the men that I had met in Boston (except they didn't *paaak the caaa*). The difference was in me. I came to the situation with a new attitude because I was in a new place.

My expectations were different and so the outcomes of my meetings with people were different. This was my first experience with the fact that you actually do get what you expect. In Boston, my experiences with men were negative because that's what I had expected. By being in a different place, I had allowed myself to have a clean slate.

Although I did not sleep with every man I went out with, I did begin to have quite a bit of sexual experience. The reason I mention this is because these experiences actually helped my self-esteem. Now freak out on me! I am not saying that sleeping around is a good way for a young woman to achieve some sense of self-worth.

Annette Mucci-Haggerty

I realize that quite a few young women actually feel worse about themselves when they give their bodies to men for the wrong reasons. They are looking for love in all of the wrong places. They use sex as a replacement for love and so end up worse off than when the started.

My situation was different in the way that I felt completely unattractive and desirable - so unattractive that I actually felt good about a man wanting me - if only for sex. What I've just told you is pitiful at best, I know, but that doesn't make it any less true. What I am saying is this: prior to Colorado, I had felt so completely ugly that it actually boosted my self-image in my mind to know that a man wanted to sleep with me at all! UGH! I know that men in Boston had wanted to sleep with me also but I had wanted them to LIKE me. I guess that I had since decided that just feeling sexy was better than feeling unloved.

Keep in mind that the reason that it didn't make me feel worse is because that somehow I was able to keep love out of the entire thing. I never slept with someone if I really wanted to hear from him ever again. In other words, if I had sex with a man I wrote him off the next day. I figured that he would think of me as "easy" and not want to take me out.

What surprised me was that some of those write offs actually did call and take me out again. No, I didn't end up long term with any of them, but I was the one who ended some of those situations. Imagine that! Not only was I chubby, I was "easy" and still they came back!

Now let me share one of my best moments. A moment that made me feel special, attractive, and wanted for one of the first times in my adult life.

There was a man named David. He worked at the company where I worked. He was the guy that all of the girls at the office wanted. He was married but he was a big flirt and everyone was trying to catch his eye. Of course, I was not immune to his charms either.

I worked a second job as a bartender at a bowling alley so I started an office bowling league. I convinced David without too much trouble that he should join the league. Once David joined, so did some of the women who were "after" him (and I got a commission for bringing a new league into the bowling alley!).

We bowled on Wednesday evenings. Afterwards most of us would land at a nearby pub for a few drinks. David always sat with me and we would talk for hours. Never once did I think he was interested in me. I knew that he liked talking to me, but come on! I was chubby, he was married (unhappily, of course) and if he did want to cheat it would be with one of the cuter women (who much to my dismay, were constantly trying to get his attention).

Then one night, David let me drive his Corvette. I was thrilled to say the least, but still did not think anything of it. After the short ride, he walked me over to my truck and once I was settled in he leaned down to say goodbye and to kiss me - I thought - on the cheek.

What happened was something that I will never forget as long as I live.

Instead of a kiss on the cheek, he planted a big, long, wet and glorious kiss on me! David - the guy who all the girls wanted - was kissing chubby, unattractive me in the parking lot! Will wonders never cease?

Now I know that you are thinking, "Come on. He was married. Just wanted a fling."

You may be right. Also, I may have been an awful person to let a married man kiss me or to even want him in the first place but at that moment I did not care one bit. In my young, confused mind the fact that he was married just made me feel more special. Here he was, choosing me to cheat on his wife with! He could have had a skinny girl, but he picked me!

Before you get too upset with me I want you to know that this did not go very far. We did make out a few times and he even took me to lunch once but it did not turn into a big "affair". I actually ended up moving back home to Boston not long afterwards. All I know is that I will always remember the time that someone was attracted to ME - the "me" inside as well as the "me" on the outside. After all, for weeks before this, we had done nothing but talk.

He had taken the time to get to know me and I will never forget him for that.

My theories

Now I will give you some tips on a new way to think. A way of thinking that will help you to be consistently nice to your body, instead of abusing it by alternately starving it and stuffing it.

I've told you to stop expecting results in a short period of time. What you should be doing, and what will keep you on track is if you:

1) *Begin thinking about how good you will look 10 years from now.*

"Now she's really gone over the edge," is probably what you are saying to yourself. "How can I give up on looking good now and think about 10 years from now? I can't stand myself for another minute *today*!" I know, it sounds like giving up, but it is far from giving up. It is giving *over*. I'm trying to say that it is acceptance of reality.

I once took a class to become certified in personal training. The instructor told us something that I will never forget because it was simple and made incredible sense. Here it is: the definition of stress is simply fighting against reality.

The reality is that it is impossible to get from overweight to thin overnight. It probably took years of thinking badly about yourself and using food as something other than fuel for you to have a visible problem. It cannot all be turned around in a short time. You can, however take a first step or maybe a couple of steps in one day, the biggest one being to look at yourself clearly. See that you are special and that in time all of the damage can be turned around. Give yourself a vacation and stop trying to rush things.

This is the best medicine to help you stick to your goals. You want to know why? The reason is because setting a goal to look better in a year or so and to FEEL better in a few days is a realistic goal. It is a do-able goal and since it is, you will not get discouraged and be inclined to give up and start over tomorrow (which will most probably take you backwards instead of forwards).

When you decide that you have to lose five pounds in a week or fit into those size seven jeans in a month, you are setting yourself up for unhealthy eating. You are giving yourself all of that ammunition to hate yourself at every little mistake.

You may, in fact fit into those jeans in a month but can you keep up the pattern? Can you continue to deprive yourself and worry about every bite of food forever? You know that is what you will have to do to stay in those jeans - so you will still have an eating problem whether you wear a size five or a size 25.

So why not try something different? What if your goal becomes just to feel better physically and better about yourself in general? This you can accomplish in a week or *as little as a few days*. What if your goal is to be healthy and to look five years younger when you are 10 years older? You will have no reason to beat yourself up at every turn! You can afford to forgive yourself because there is no rush. You are after good health not a smaller pair of jeans. If this approach over time just happens to improve your appearance (and make no mistake - it will) well, who are you to complain?

2) Stop comparing yourself to other skinny, in-shape people.

It's OK to Eat
Be Fit, Healthy, and NOT on a Diet

Every time you compare yourself to someone who is thinner, prettier (in your opinion) or healthier than you are it makes you feel bad. Feeling bad is what got you into this mess. After all, feeling as if you are inadequate in any way at all makes you dislike yourself. Disliking yourself can lead to all sorts of nastiness.

One such nasty thing might be creating an emptiness that screams to be filled. Unfortunately you don't think that you have what is required to fill this need - I think that we can safely name this as the need to feel special, to be loved. So you try to fill your emptiness by stuffing yourself. You tell yourself that you are hungry for food, when in fact you are hungry for love.

Another issue here is about self-fulfilling prophecy. If you make up your mind that you are unattractive, is it possible that you may actually be trying unconsciously to make sure that you ARE unattractive and stay that way? Is it possible that even though you hate feeling unattractive and overweight, you are used to this feeling and it feels safer than the alternative? Or that you have to prove yourself right by keeping up the image?

You start eating and then you feel another need. This is the need to punish yourself for being so weak as to be putting food in your mouth when you think that you should be doing just the opposite. Well, what better way to punish yourself than to eat more food and then you can call yourself names and tell yourself that you are an awful fat cow (after all, look at all of those skinny people who aren't so weak as you) and so the cycle continues.

Again, I will remind you that I myself lived this cycle of self-hatred and abuse so I know how it feels.

Well, what if you did the opposite? What if you started opening your eyes to all of the people (and there are quite a lot, unfortunately) who are *heavier* than you or the people who aren't as pretty as you - or as smart as you? Then maybe you would begin to see that **you aren't so bad as you think that you are.**

Then *look very closely* at those supposedly beautiful people whom you may have decided are better than you. Are they really so perfect? I used to think that the definition of beautiful was thin. That was it. If someone was thin, then they were beautiful and I wanted to be them. I certainly didn't want to be myself, now did I?

Then I began to change my thinking and to look a bit closer. Well, that one is very thin, yes but her thighs still jiggle when she walks - just like mine do.

That lucky devil is probably three sizes smaller than me, but look at the rolls of loose flesh on her stomach!

Now **there** is someone who does have a nice body, but she wears so much make up its scary and her skin is terrible!

That's not even counting the people who were more out of shape and larger than I was!

Now don't get your blood pressure in an uproar over this! I am in no way suggesting that you begin to make *fun* of anybody. I am not even suggesting that you voice your opinions out loud. Most of all, I am *absolutely not* suggesting that you begin to think that you are better than any of these people.

What I am suggesting is that you stop looking around comparing yourself only to models on the cover of magazines and famous actresses (and even on them, you can see things that aren't perfect). What I am suggesting is that you begin to realize that **no one is better than you.**

Just stop comparing yourself to impossibly thin people. Even if you look at thin people, notice that they are not perfect either. If you don't believe me, ask them. I'm sure one of them will tell you. I'll just bet that if you were to walk up to the most beautiful girl you can find and tell her that you think that she is perfect she will say "thank-you" and then launch right into a list of all of the things that she thinks is wrong with her. Sad but true.

By starting to think in the opposite way that you have been, you will start to bear witness to your own specialness - your own attractiveness. I believe that you cannot treat yourself well if you don't see that you are wonderful in your own right and that you deserve to be treated as such. (Something I unfortunately had to learn by having a married man kissing me!)

The makers of most diet products show us small beautiful women that we want to emulate. By doing this, they only make us feel more unworthy which is exactly the opposite of the way we should feel. They convince us that we can look so much better in no time at all. It is only that we are eating the wrong stuff, using the wrong diets, not exercising enough. That is why we are fat and unattractive. These diet sellers want us to believe that it is just a physical thing, like acne or some other skin disease. It has nothing to do with our self-esteem or lack thereof.

What I decided to try when I had enough of the diet-go-round was thinking the opposite way. Maybe I should look at people and see that they also have physical faults so that I could see that yes, I was no better - but neither was I worse than anyone else.

Maybe I should start looking at myself and pointing out my attributes instead of all of my faults.

Okay, so I did have a very large behind and even larger thighs, but I also always had a waist no matter how much weight I gained. Yes, I couldn't wear anything I wanted to wear but I was smart enough to know what I shouldn't be caught dead in, unlike a lot of women (even those who were smaller than me) out there. (Let me point out here that there are very few people that look good in just about anything). I may not have been the most beautiful woman in the world but my skin was good and I knew how not to overload my face with gobs of make-up.

I knew that when I wanted to be, I could be charming and people could like me (at least when I had the courage to be outgoing and let them see my personality). I loved doing nice things for people and that was something, wasn't it?

These thoughts made me feel better about myself. Then when I was of a mind to stuff myself (and so stuff all of my emotional pain) maybe I could give myself a reason to slow down. I started to try to think like an already thin person instead of a fat person. People always say that they wish that they could eat whatever they wanted to. Well, think about this: people without a food problem *do* eat whatever they want to. **They just don't want to eat everything.**

Now, the next thing I want to tell you about- and this is, I think, the most difficult thing of all.

3) You must learn to forgive yourself.

What prompts us to keep repeating the cycle? I'm talking about the cycle that our Betty in the first chapter was living. The one where you try to diet, screw up just a little bit and then decide to eat everything that doesn't run as fast as you do. You do this because after all, you've ruined today and you are probably going to eat nothing at all tomorrow to make up for it so you might as well eat all of the things that you will soon be deprived of… NOW!

It is that little voice inside of us that tells us that we have failed, we are a loser, we screwed up the whole day and so why even bother? If we really listen to that stinking little voice we will let it call us names (*stupid, worthless, fat, lazy*) and go on to tell us that we will probably never succeed. We will always be fat and unattractive so why not just accept it? We allow ourselves to beat our*selves* up -unforgiving and relentlessly torturing our spirits because we ate a cookie! Berating ourselves because we are hungry and want to eat anything at all.

Food becomes the enemy when in fact (now listen to this and listen to this good) **food is a requirement of life**. It is a necessity and God or whomever you believe in put it here in order for us to live. **Everyone has the right to eat**.

Here is what you have to do to shut that nasty voice up for good. You have to stop playing that awful, abusive tape in your head and come up with an entirely new tape. Put a new voice on a new tape that tells you that there is no shame in being hungry and *<u>absolutely no shame in eating</u>*. Food was put on this planet for us to eat and enjoy and feeling guilty for eating it is just

It's OK to Eat
Be Fit, Healthy, and NOT on a Diet

plain silly. Does a cow or a dog ever feel guilty for eating? Do they worry about how much they ate and try to starve themselves the next day to make up for it? No, of course not.

Okay. Dogs are dogs and we are people but the concept is still the same. We need food to survive. Food tastes wonderful. Why shouldn't we enjoy it?

Would you ever do something so mean to your kids as to give them clothes to wear (a necessity of life, as is food) and then try to make them feel guilty and ashamed for wearing them? No, of course not! So why should you be ashamed of being hungry and wanting to eat? No reason I can think of. When your children are hungry, you feed them.

Now there is scientific proof that your body's metabolism speeds up and slows down according to what you put into it. For example, if you eat when you are hungry and keep a constant supply of food going to your body whenever it is necessary, your metabolism will constantly work at its comfortable speed. If you eat extra food, your metabolism will then speed up (or burn more fat faster) in order to get rid of the extra food so it can stay at its comfortable weight. If you keep eating extra food for a prolonged period however (I'm talking weeks here), your body will get used to this and settle back into its normal speed.

Now, what happens when you eat less food or hardly any food? Your body thinks that it is starving and your metabolism *slows down* (burns off less fat) because it wants to keep you from starving to death. So starving yourself is not really a good idea because then when you eat any thing at all, your body will actually try to store as much of the fat as possible to keep you alive.

Your hunger will also increase and decrease over time according to how your lifestyle and movements change. I can illustrate this by sharing with you something that I recently went through.

I had been teaching nine aerobics classes per week, continuously for about a year. Then I started a new job and I had to decrease my aerobics schedule. I cut down to four classes per week and began sitting for longer hours than I was used to.

After a month or so, I noticed that my pants were getting uncomfortable and I was feeling a bit bloated. What was going on here? I began to get a bit panicky. I knew that teaching less would tend to make me burn less fat, but I was still eating only when hungry so why were my clothes getting smaller? I was worried that I was going to become a fat person again and considered whether I should actually start watching my fat grams and counting calories.

NO WAY! The smart side of my brain told me. No matter how tempting it seemed I couldn't get back on that "diet-go-round" ever again. I decided to hold off on the panic, and wait this whole situation out. After all, even though my pants were a bit tight, I still looked okay in my stretchy aerobics clothes and with no clothes on at all.

Instead of dieting, I bought myself some new pants made with stretchy fabric. At least I could be comfortable. Notice that I never weighed myself.

Doesn't matter how much I weigh, only how my clothes fit and how I feel about myself.

The final outcome of this story is this: in a few months, I was back to normal. Looking back I can see clearly what had happened. I cut down my classes but at first my body didn't know that I wasn't going be moving around as much and burning as much fuel. My very intelligent body kept me hungry enough to eat enough to keep me going so at first I was eating more than I needed. After a time, my body began to realize that I had slowed down somewhat and my appetite diminished. It didn't happen overnight so I didn't really notice it as it was happening.

Now, however, I can see that I don't get as hungry as often as I used to and that is fine with me. I spend less money on food this way! The wonderful point here is that this proves just how the whole thing works, *if you pay attention to your actual hunger and have a little faith.*

Notice something else important here. I was eating the same amount after I slowed down my workouts,

It's OK to Eat
Be Fit, Healthy, and NOT on a Diet

but I didn't start to gain anything until a *whole month* went by. This proves that one or two days of pigging out will not make a difference.

So let's put this theory into work. Let's say you have been eating in a healthier way and one day you lose it and eat everything in sight. You start to feel bad about yourself and the tape starts to play in your head full blast. Now is when you can concentrate on playing the new tape.

It should sound something like this: *I will not feel guilty for something I ate. There is nothing wrong with eating and I will trust my body to do its job and take care of the excess. One day of extra food does **not** make a person go up a size. I work hard. I am a good mother (wife, sister, friend, whatever) and I am an awesome, beautiful, special person. I deserve to eat and enjoy my food. I will let this go and NOT try to make up for it by starving tomorrow. Starving tomorrow will only make my situation worse, as it has in the past. I am going to have the courage to do this a* *new way. I believe that eating is natural and my body will take care of itself.*

This will take some getting used to. It is not easy to shut that old voice on that very old tape up. It will keep at you, but you can just keep answering it back. Write the whole thing down if you have to. I still, after almost 10 years of thinking like this, have to remind myself once in a while. I have not yet succeeded in killing that stinking voice completely.

But remember this: **you can shut that voice up and replace it with a new and kind voice.**

4

What To Think About When You Want To Eat

My Story

I lived in Denver for just a bit over three years. I came back to Boston about 20 pounds thinner than when I had left although I was still a bit heavy for my height. I was probably a size 11 by that time and was still riding the diet roller coaster, thinking about food all of the time. I finally felt strong enough to come home and face my fears about the people in Boston. I had realized that my very own vision of who I was in reality shaped others image of me. They saw what I saw. So maybe it was time that I should see something different. Something *better*.

While living on my own I got the foundations necessary for me to learn that I was indeed special and to begin to love myself. What I had gained was the beginnings of self-confidence. I had begun to think myself worth something and weight had nothing whatsoever to do with it. Most people think (I was guilty of this myself) that if they can just get thin, if they can just get beautiful then they can start to love themselves. It doesn't work that way. It's the opposite. **If you can just learn to love yourself, then you can get thin** - and stay that way.

Let me share with you one of the things that helped me to learn this invaluable lesson.

I used to go clubbing with a girl who was skinny, blonde, cute, dressed nice - you name it. She was what I would have thought any man would want. Here were the two of us-her in her killer outfits with the nice little fanny and me in my full skirts which were all that I could wear to sufficiently cover my own extremely ample fanny.

After a few months of being out in Denver, I had begun to let my*self* show. I became outgoing and friendly and decided not to be afraid to talk to anyone, even the most gorgeous cowboy (oh, how I loved those cowboy boots).

An amazing thing began to happen. More and more often, it was *me* who went home with my phone number in some guy's pocket. *No way!* How could this be? Could it be that I was attractive even though I was chunky? Could it be that I had a fun personality and someone would choose to take me out over my skinny friend? WOW! It turns out that even though my friend was attractive and did in fact have a fun personality, she used to just stand there leaning against the bar with a look of (bitchy?) contempt on her face that pretty much put the men off. I, on the other hand, was friendly, outgoing and (so I'd been told) fun to talk to.

After learning some new lessons about self-confidence, I came home to work at the family ice-cream business in order to pay off some debt. I was planning to move back to Denver at the end of the summer. As it turned out, I never made it.

You see, on Labor Day weekend I met the man that I ended up marrying.

I had lost more weight by that time. I was actually down to a loose size 5 but had to face the reality that I still couldn't wear short shorts and spandex because even though my bulges were much smaller, they were sill bulges. I had yet to learn the power of exercise.

I also learned a couple of other lessons that were imperative for me to grow.

Annette Mucci-Haggerty

One was that I could actually make my dreams come true. I had always - since I had first become aware that I was a chubby teenager - had a vision of being skinny, tanned, driving a sports car and having a handsome boyfriend. Having a REAL boyfriend was difficult for me. I had gone out with lots of men, but only a couple of them prior to age 24 could I call my boyfriend.

Now here I was cruising up the highway, tanned and in my tight little jeans, driving my Mazda Rx-7 on the way to my boyfriend's house. A boyfriend who just happened to be an ex jock, captain of his high school and college football team and someone who I could never have "gotten" in high school.

That was the good part. For the first time in my life I was able to experience the feeling of making a vision actually become real. It was something that I had thought was possible for other people, but never for me. It was awesome.

But why then, wasn't I happy? I had all of the ingredients that I had thought were required to be positively giddy at age 24 and still I wasn't happy.

Hence the second lesson. Maybe there was more to being happy than just being thin? Maybe all of the things I had blamed on being fat didn't have anything to do with being fat?

The third lesson was just as important. It was this. I was thin, no denying that. But I was obnoxious thin. I was that person I mentioned in the first chapter - counting every bite of food I put in my mouth and bragging to people (I had actually thought that they'd be interested. Can you believe it?) that I had only eaten 2 bites of this and 3 bites of that and wasn't I doing well?

I was thin, yes, but I was obsessed with food. I was obsessed with keeping track all of the food that I was eating and counting all of the food that I was denying myself. Imagine someone who was supposed to be so happy doing such work on a daily basis? I was waking up congratulating myself on going to bed hungry the night before. Now that was a successful day! Oh YAY!

My huge days were behind me (not counting being pregnant) but it wasn't until much later that I learned how not to have a food problem.

By now you are probably asking, "That's it? There must be more to it than this! What did she eat? When did she eat? How did she lose all of that weight?" I dieted, of course. I starved myself. What do you think? "Well," you might think, "at least she was successful in losing that fat!"

Success? I don't think so. Not yet, anyway.

My Theories

Here are some ideas to help you when you want to eat.

1) *Listen to your body.*

"What does this have to do with eating?" you ask. Everything!

How many times have you eaten for no other reason than you were depressed, happy, bored, or just because some diet you were trying to follow told you that it was time to eat? Not one of these reasons is a good reason for chowing down. There is only one good reason to eat.

A person should eat only because he or she is hungry. This seems simple doesn't it? But as you know, it is not simple at all.

It's OK to Eat
Be Fit, Healthy, and NOT on a Diet

We have been eating for all of the wrong reasons for so long that we have forgotten how to tell if we are actually hungry. After all, whenever we eat we are usually convinced that we are hungry when in fact we are not. Food ends up being used to heal wounds, to reward ourselves or to punish ourselves.

Think back. How long has it been since you have actually eaten only because you were just plain hungry? Or skipped a meal because you just *weren't* hungry? (yes, that can happen). How long since you have based your decision of what to eat on exactly what you were craving instead of what you thought was the "right" thing to eat?

This is my advice to you. Start to really focus on your body's messages. *Wait.*

Think about your stomach and how it *feels*. ***Wait***. Don't eat just because it's breakfast time and some expert told you that it was bad to skip breakfast. WAIT.

My goodness, don't we realize how awesome each of our bodies is and that it can take care of such things? Did our infant children suck a bottle or our breast when they weren't hungry? Didn't they do just fine when they didn't eat much for a couple of days because they were sick? (If you have kids, you know how impossible it is to make them eat when they don't want to).

Learn to FEEL. Every time you think you want to eat ask yourself why. Am I really hungry? Am I trying to fill some need other than hunger? Maybe you are trying to stuff some bad feelings. Maybe you just have to learn to sit still and just *feel bad.*

I'm serious about this. We all run around like little chickens when we feel bad, shopping, eating, partying - anything to avoid feeling bad. Maybe the best way to handle feeling bad is just to sit still and feel bad and get it over with instead of stuffing food down our throats which is only going to make us feel worse.

Now this next part is important. If you decide that you are in fact legitimately hungry then you go right ahead and eat. You have the green light. If you should decide that you are not actually hungry yet, then try putting off eating until you are. Don't tell yourself that you can't eat at all, only that you have to wait until you are hungry.

Part two to listening to your body (I think that this is a bit harder to do) is to **stop eating when you are full.** Let me stipulate that I am not saying *stuffed*, I am saying *full* - or even better, simply no longer hungry.

What I did when I was starting my new attitudes towards food was to literally pause in-between every bite and question how I felt. This takes practice but after a while it will happen naturally. Ask yourself: *Am I still hungry? Or am I just going to take another bite because it tastes good? Am I worried about wasting food?* Because there is no worse way of wasting food than to shove it into a body that doesn't need it.

Let me say this again in another way because this is extremely important. It is still the same waste of food if you throw it away or of you eat it when you don't need it. **Eating food that you don't need is like turning your body into a dumpster.**

A wonderful tool to help you to stop eating when you are full is called a "doggy bag". We've all heard of it. We need to use it more often.

Again, it is always okay to eat if you are genuinely hungry. If you are full and you really want to eat the rest because it tastes good or you don't want to waste the food well then take it home! Tell yourself that of course you can eat the rest, you just *can't eat it right now* because it would be a waste if you did.

What will happen if you stick to stopping when you are full is that the answer to that question (whether to keep eating or not) will become clearer all of the time. You will get more in touch with your body and you will be able to stop more easily - especially if you keep your promise to yourself that you can, in fact have the rest later when you get hungry again. Also, your tolerance to that bloated overstuffed feeling will decrease. It will get to the point that you just can't stand to feel that full. This, like everything else I've mentioned will not happen over night but it WILL HAPPEN eventually if you keep trying.

2) Never allow yourself to feel guilty while eating!!!!!!

This one, in case you couldn't tell from the exclamation points is a really big one. I know that I have already mentioned guilt in a previous chapter. This time it's a bit different. What I talked about before was the guilt you feel *after* you eat. Now, I'm talking about the guilt you feel *while* eating.

Guilt while eating sabotages the entire experience. We eat because we are hungry, yes, but it is certainly all right to enjoy eating. Food tastes wonderful, does it not? Food nourishes us and gives us what our body needs to grow and stay healthy.

So why in heaven should we feel guilty about it?

That, however is just what people with food problems do. We feel guilty even while we are eating. This is a serious problem because it causes more eating, which then causes more guilt. You can see where I'm going with this.

If you are eating some delicious morsel and the whole time you are saying things to yourself like: "*I should not be eating this. This is going to make me fat and I'm already fat enough. What is wrong with me? I can't seem to say "NO" to anything! I will just have to starve myself for the rest of the day to make up for this,*" (sound familiar?) all that you are going to accomplish with this train of thought is that you will not enjoy your food. If you don't enjoy your food then you will not end your eating experience feeling satisfied. If you do not feel satisfied with what you just ate then *you will most certainly be looking for something else to eat as soon as possible.*

You know the rest of that story. You eat again and feel even more guilt the next time and so the torture cycle continues.

My question is this: Why put yourself through all of that? Why not enjoy your food guilt free and have done with it? I actually have been known to moan during eating.

After I am done I say to myself (literally), "That was delicious. I deserved that." Then I forget about it until I get hungry again.

This leads me right into my next bit of advice.

3) *Enjoy your food as much as possible.*

It goes to follow that by not allowing yourself to feel guilty while eating you will end up actually enjoying your food. This is a big plus. After all, if we didn't care about taste and enjoyment then we would just eat grain and rice all of the time. We would just have a hole in our sides or somewhere that we could fill up with swill from a hose. Flavor wouldn't matter.

So when you are sitting in front of that beautiful piece of steak, allow yourself to savor it. Take a big whiff before you take a bite. Put that bite into your mouth and just chew it nice and slowly and really *taste* it. Let those delicious juices flow and MMMMM, just enjoy.

What is this going to accomplish? You will feel a whole lot more satisfied when you are finished, that's what. If you feel satisfied that your eating experience was wonderful then maybe there won't be as much of a hurry to go do it again right away. I'm sure I don't need to tell you that a delicious eating experience rushed and stuffed will result in those awful feelings of disgust in yourself that I've mentioned before.

It is your choice. You can stuff your food, feeling guilty and anxious all the while and end up eating more than you need or really want. This will result in pain and shame (if you let it). Or you can eat slowly and love every minute of it and stop when you are full and end your eating experience feeling satisfied and good about the whole thing.

I don't think that this is a difficult choice to make.

Which brings me to the next important issue.

4) *Concentrate intensely on how you feel when you overeat.*

You have to know that it will take time to get to the point where you can just eat whatever you want and it will turn out to not be too much. Old habits take time to break. Eventually if you treat yourself well and stop abusing your emotional and physical body you will be able to chill and just let the whole eating thing happen.

Until that time you need to pay close attention to how you feel when you do eat too much. I'm not talking about torturing yourself with guilt. We've already gone over that. What I'm talking about is to just sit still and *feel physically crappy,* which is how you tend to feel when you've stuffed yourself. Think long and hard about how your stomach feels bloated (and maybe aches), how you wish you could just puke and get it all out. Think about how your waistband is tighter, how sitting down is not fun when your stomach is bloated.

Now, I want you to try to do this *without judging yourself.* In other words, observe how lousy it feels to be that full without all of the guilt and name-calling. I just want you to remember it so that next time you are eating something wonderful, you will do what I've mentioned before - stop between each bite and think. Decide if it would be better to eat it now or to wait until later so that you won't have to end up feeling this way.

Do you see what I'm getting at? Your are probably saying to yourself, "What is she talking about? Of course I know what it feels like to be full!" However, usually when we feel that way we concentrate on how "bad" we were for eating so much instead just looking at it objectively and teaching ourselves that this feeling is not fun.

A good way to look at it is this: let's say that I walk down the stairs too fast and crack my knee on the wall because I couldn't stop in time. I don't call myself names and beat myself up just because I hurt myself, do I? I don't think that I am a bad person for rushing. Nope! I would more likely just decide something like: Gee, this is not fun to bang my knee. It hurts! I think that it would be better NOT to run down the stairs again so that I can avoid this pain.

5

Practical Advice for When You Are Ready to Eat

My Story

I remember how uncomfortable it was to be fat -

Not just the emotional discomfort but also the physical discomfort. From the time I was a teenager and had discovered my chubbiness, I would not wear shorts or a bathing suit in the summer. Even in 100-degree weather I would be seen in a pair of jeans and a halter-top. I gained most of my weight on my bottom so it was safe to bare my stomach and shoulders.

I remember going shopping for pants, trying on no less than 25 pairs of jeans, shopping for hours and still leaving the mall without a single pair of pants that looked good on me. I am short and so the proportions of the jeans that were big enough for my thighs were way too big for my waist. They were made for girls much taller than me, who were naturally bigger in the trunk area.

I remember after I had my license how I would go out in the evening by myself only to end up at McDonald's buying a quarter-pounder, large fry, and an apple pie. Then I would park in an empty parking lot on the way home and suck it all down because I was embarrassed for my parents to know that I was eating an entire meal less than an hour after dinner. I don't think that I ever tasted that food because I ate it so fast.

I remember how tight my jeans were. These days I cannot stand anything to dig into me even a tiny bit but back then all I would wear were tight jeans. There were a few reasons for this. One was that the tight jeans sort of acted as a girdle and kept everything from bouncing around when I moved. Another reason was that if a pair of pants fit my waist, they were most certainly tight in the thighs. The last reason was because when I was at my biggest, I simply would not buy a size 15 pant so I wore a painfully tight size 13.

It's OK to Eat
Be Fit, Healthy, and NOT on a Diet

I remember how I used to have to lay on my back so that I could get my pants zipped and the cuts that I would get on the sides of my fingers from the zipper pulls. I can't tell you how many times those zippers just broke - just pulled away from the teeth from the constant stress. Sometimes it would even happen when I was out somewhere and I would have the humiliation of trying to get out of there and home with no one becoming aware of my predicament.

I remember in the summer when it was hot and I was working in an office wearing dresses and nylons how I would end up with chafing between my thighs from the constant rubbing when I walked. I would have to keep baby powder in my purse and constantly apply it when I was in the ladies' room.

I remember how often I had to buy new shoes. I wore high heels all of the time. I didn't even own a pair of sneakers, the theory being that if I was taller then I would appear somewhat less wide. If you have built up fat in-between your legs then you are unable to walk with your skeleton in the correct position. In other words, that fat would keep my knees from touching so I would actually have to walk with my legs spread apart to some extent. This would result in the wearing down of the insides of the soles and the heels of my shoes. If after a few months of wear, if I were to take my shoes off and try to stand them up, they would lean almost completely over into each other.

I remember working at the family ice cream joint and making myself these tiny little 3-ounce sundaes so that I could satisfy my craving without eating too much. The problem was that in one day I could eat as many as 20 of those sundaes. I remember the shame I felt then.

I remember my sides literally aching from all of the food that I had stuffed into my body and still not being able to say no to the next thing that was tempting me.

I remember waking up in the morning, dreading getting dressed. I would lie in bed and just wish that I could stay in for the whole day and not have to be faced with putting on clothes and going out. You see, I never knew if my clothes would be more uncomfortable than they were the day before - or if they would fit at all.

I remember sitting uncomfortably most of the time (pants too tight - seats of the chairs too small).

I remember going up and down stairs. What a pain!

I remember being miserable.

My Theories

Now for some more help when faced with the prospect of eating. These are all of the tricks I taught myself when I was on the road to getting rid of my food problem.

1) Put off eating a craved item.

Never say to yourself that you can never again have a… cookie, candy bar, McDonald's hamburger. If you are craving something then tell yourself that yes you can have it - later on.

This is a good method to help you distinguish between a real desire for something special to eat and a desire to abuse yourself. If you find yourself wanting a doughnut because you saw someone else eating one then you can say to yourself, "I can most definitely have a doughnut but I think I'll just wait until later when I am really hungry. That way I will enjoy it so much more."

One of two things will happen. When you do get legitimately hungry you will find that you would rather eat something more substantial than a doughnut (something with some vitamins, perhaps?). Or, two - you will still be dying to eat that doughnut. If you are, then by all means go for it.

As you know, I used to have a weakness for a McDonalds number 3 (quarter pounder-with cheese, fry) super-sized with a diet coke. I would eat that food twice a day if I could. Then I started telling myself that yes, I could have my number 3. No Problem.

TOMORROW.

Sometimes tomorrow would come and my overwhelming desire would be much less. Then I would tell myself to try and wait another day. Other times I would wait the day and find that yes, I HAD to have my quarter-pounder with cheese and that was that. If that was the case than that is what I would do. Eat it and enjoy every bite of it.

Of course, I would use all of my other skills while fulfilling my desire: not eating at all until I was good and hungry, stopping when I was full and not feeling the least bit guilty during or after eating.

There is an important element to this skill. **Never lie to yourself**.

If you tell yourself that you can have a candy bar later only to deny yourself when you find that you still want it then you will be back at square one, won't you? Basically you will be saying that you can *never* have it and that will make the desire all the more powerful until it overcomes you and you eat a dozen candy bars. Not to mention the fact that putting things off will never work for you because you will know inside that you are really trying to not eat it at all. This will most likely lead to even more binging. So when you make promises to yourself, keep them. The more you tell yourself the truth, the more this tool will help you.

Let me explain at this point that changing your mind and deciding that you didn't really want the candy bar that badly after all is not the same as lying. If you were legitimately hungry and still desiring the candy bar then you could have it. Maybe in the time that has passed you have started desiring something else entirely.

2) Try taking just one bite of something that you are having trouble putting off or saying no to.

This technique is extremely helpful when someone is eating something delicious in front of you and you know that you are really not hungry. You should first try to do the previous thing. Try to put it off until later.

Sometimes this will just not do it for you. That hot fudge sundae just looks so good and you really want the taste of that in your mouth. I suggest that you ask your friend for a bite. If he or she is any kind of friend he or she will give you that bite. That should do it.

My theory is this. There are times when you just need a taste of something. You just want to stimulate those buds with whatever is haunting us at the moment. Most likely you really do not even want the whole thing. If you are at the place where you are allowing yourself these small pleasures and not beating yourself up for wanting them, then there should be no problem in taking a bite, savoring it and saying, "Thank you. That's just what I needed."

Now, it may turn out that you want more. Well then if you are not in fact truly hungry you can just promise yourself that in an hour or two, when you become hungry then you will just march yourself back to that particular ice-cream place and have yourself a sundae. Or if it was a candy bar, you will pull that sucker right out of your pocket and have at it. No problem, right? No one is telling you that you can't *ever* have it.

On the other hand, I have found for myself that there are many times that it is my mouth that wants the chocolate cake and if I go buy a whole piece only to find out that I really didn't want the whole thing, then I will eat the whole thing anyway. After all, I don't want to waste it!

Well, here's what to do if that should happen to you. If you find that you bought something that you find you didn't really want as much as you thought you did and it turns out to be something that you can't save for later, **throw it away**. Maybe you just had to buy it to prove to yourself that you could have it if you wanted to and no one was going to stop you. You took your one or two bites and then you find that you just can't eat it because you are not hungry enough to feel good about it.

I hate to waste food as much as anybody else but you have to *throw it away*. That's right. Toss it. You may be able to find someone to give it to but rather than eat it, TOSS IT. Remember, it is just as much a waste of food to eat something that you don't need as it is to throw it away. Chalk it up to a lesson well learned and maybe next time you won't buy it at all. **Make sure that you don't feel guilty about it**. You already know where that leads.

3) If you are enjoying one of those rare times that you are, in fact hungry but not desiring anything special then, chose the healthy thing.

Let's say that you are getting the hang of this whole not-eating-unless-you-are-really-hungry routine.

Let's say that your stomach is growling but you really can't decide what it is that you actually want to eat. Well, this is the time that you MUST try to choose the healthy thing.

Have a salad with grilled chicken (delicious, actually) or some meat and broccoli. I love to put marinara sauce on my broccoli - especially if I'm having it with chicken Parmesan. By the way, broccoli is a great substitute for pasta.

What I'm getting at is this. Save the big splurges for when you really need them, like when you are craving something awful (I should say awfully good) or when you just don't have the time to eat the right thing. If you are fortunate enough to be in one of those lovely situations where you don't care what it is as long as you fill that spot in your belly then take advantage of the situation. Eat something healthy.

Notice that I am not preaching about eating non-fat or low calorie here. I am not even sure that I would agree that everything non-fat is necessarily good for you. I'm just talking about eating something healthy - something with fiber and protein and vitamins.

It will probably still be delicious and you may find yourself actually craving healthy stuff before long. If you had told me that there would come a day when I would go out of my way for some seasoned green beans from the Chinese place up the street I would have told you that you were certifiable. However, I am happy to say that I actually have been known to do just that!

Keep in mind that it is obviously not my intention to put you on a diet. Nor am I recommending any diet at all. You have tried plenty of them. You know what is good for you. You know what isn't. You know if a lot of carbohydrates make you feel bloated (they do me). You know if dairy products bother your stomach (they don't bother me). It is not my intention to tell you what to eat. It is my intention to help you to choose and to eat better.

4) Practice leaving at least one bite on your plate.

This will help you get you to the place where you can stop eating when you are full. If you are currently in the habit of cleaning your plate then you can ease into not eating it all by leaving just one bite (and make it a reasonable sized bite) all of the time. You can gradually increase to two bites, then three and so on. It really will get easier and eventually you will be able to leave as much as is necessary. This works.

In fact, after some time of practicing leaving food on your plate and listening to your stomach to see if you are truly hungry before taking another bite, your tolerance for feeling bloated will decrease. I am to the point where most of the time I know exactly when to stop without even thinking about it. I just *know* that if I take one more bite it will put me over the edge and I will feel stuffed. I hate that stuffed feeling. Look at the difference: I used to eat entire meals when I already felt stuffed. Now I can rarely eat even one bite!

5) *Don't forget about your doggie bags.*

It is always easier to tell yourself you can finish it later than to tell yourself that you just can't finish it at all. Take the leftovers home and when you get hungry again, most certainly go ahead and enjoy them. This can also save a lot of money on lunches the next day!

6) *Eat your vegetables first.*

I grew up in a house where the only vegetables I ever ate were potatoes and corn. I had to develop a taste for broccoli and carrots and green beans, etc after I grew up and moved out. Now I can't believe I sometimes actually *crave vegetables*. Will wonders never cease!!

What I do when I have a meal is to eat a few bites of my veggies first (this does not include French fries!) This way I make sure I get my fiber and I also fill up a bit before getting to the meat. I recommend keeping the starch (empty calories that act like paste in your bowels) until last. Again, don't tell yourself that you can't have them, take a few bites and decide to leave most of them until the end. Hopefully, if you've mastered stopping when full you will by this time have no room left for them. End result is that you are eating your veggies (fiber) and your meat (protein).

I actually learned a trick to get rid of most of my potato and pasta eating problems by accident. A friend of mine, Gretchen (who is a size 2, I think) told me about the way that she eats to avoid getting bloated. I honestly don't know the diet or the specific rules but the jist of it is that it's not good to mix your proteins and your carbohydrates.

The thinking is that your body doesn't digest your food properly if you are putting too much different stuff into it at the same time. What you should do, according to Gretchen is to eat your protein and then wait about 3 hours until you have totally digested and then you can eat your carbs. Apparently, it is okay to eat your veggies (not potatoes because they are a starch) with your protein but not pasta or rice etc. Again, I'm not recommending this particular diet, only telling you what Gretchen does and how I learned from it.

Anyway, I hung around with Gretchen for a while and saw that she ate plenty but never gained any weight so I decided that I could try this thing to a certain extent. I decided that I could not ever live without French fries or spaghetti (been down that road) but that I could probably eat my steak and broccoli and save the French fries for later.

What ended up happening was that I lived without the French fries because I enjoyed my veggies and meat so much that I ended up forgetting about the fries altogether. I'm not even speculating about whether Gretchen's diet works or not but I do know that I am much less bloated when I don't eat so many carbs. Plus things move through me so much better when I eat my veggies if you catch my meaning.

Which leads me to my next point.

7) *Fiber.*

Fiber is important because it helps to clean you out. Did you ever wonder how that fat that you end up losing gets out of your body? Fiber, that's how. Fiber absorbs fat and carries that fat out with it through your bowels.

Without getting into too much of a discussion about poop here, let me mention one more thing. If you are having trouble with your movements, then you might want to do a bowel cleanse. A bowel cleanse is where you drink a lot of fluids and eat lots of fiber for a couple of days to give your plumbing a good cleaning out. An herb called Cascara Sagrada can help with this (remember, I'm not a physician so don't do anything without doctor's permission). Has it occurred to you that any clogging of the works can slow down everything else - by this I mean digestion, metabolism, etc? You definitely want to keep things moving if you want to be healthy, feel better and to get smaller in size.

I feel that it is important that I mention that I am not advising you to use bowel movements as a way to get rid of food that you may feel that you shouldn't have eaten. I myself went through that stage when I was younger when I would take Ex-lax hoping that I could get the food out of me quicker and make up for the fact that I ate it at all. (I never could make myself puke so this was my version of bulimia, I guess).

I'm speaking here of maintenance. I'm talking about keeping things cleaned out and working properly for health reasons. Plus, it just feels better to get rid of the excess. I am NOT talking about abusing any substance that makes your bowels move in order to make up for overeating. I've already talked about letting your body take care of itself in that respect.

8) *Make your goals small and make a big deal out of those small victories.*

You have already tried to make those drastic changes time and time again. You have told yourself that you are going to go on this starvation diet and stick with it forever. You have put unbelievable pressures on yourself and then beaten yourself up when you couldn't stick with them. Let me ask you this, where did that get you? Why not make small, doable goals for yourself and congratulate yourself when you are successful?

I will give you an example of this from my own experience. I discovered that a slice of cheese had six grams of fat in it. Six grams of fat in one little slice of cheese! There were two slices of cheese on one quarter-pounder alone! Imagine if I just gave up cheese.

I could still have the burger, but I would just go without the cheese. I did the math and decided that I probably ate at least five slices of cheese per week, which would total 30 grams of fat. In one year, I would probably eat somewhere around *1500 fewer grams of fat*! WOW!

That seemed very doable to me and you know what? It was. It surprised me how good the burgers and ham sandwiches etc still tasted without the cheese. As a matter of fact, the cheese sort of took away from the taste of the meat.

I did it. I felt good.

There were other small victories that all added up to bigger ones. They worked. I could keep with these little sacrifices because they were not all at once life altering. Plus, don't forget I had already given up on the old Overnight Thinking. I wanted to be healthy and good to my body and look good when I'm 50, so I could live with these small changes.

Now look at me.

So let's recap. I put off eating my fries until I digested my meat. I ended up not eating the fries at all. Now when I get a burger and fries, I do eat some fries but not even half of the box. They just are not a big deal to me. Besides, I can eat them whenever I want to so what's the rush? I have a feeling McDonald's is not going to go out of business anytime soon so there will always be plenty of fries out there for me.

I managed for over a year to leave off the cheese but now I find that I don't have to anymore. I usually only eat about half of a burger anyway so it doesn't matter. (Don't forget that if I'm really hungry, I have no problem cleaning my plate). I'm eating a lot less stuff but also with a lot less hardship. Let me remind you, I didn't try to make all of these changes in one day. I made them over months or even years. But I've gotten a lot further along the healthy body path in the past 10 years than I ever did throughout the first 18 or so years of my weight struggle.

Do you think that it might just be because I had stopped struggling?

Annette Mucci-Haggerty

6

Exercise: What You May Or May Not Want to Know

My Story

A funny thing happened to me after my son was born almost 8 years ago. Actually, the seeds for this occurring were probably planted over the prior years but finally that little *click* happened in my mind and everything changed. (It has been my experience that those huge life changing ideas rarely happen with fireworks but instead something in there just *clicks* - much like turning on a light).

I had tried to exercise a few times before during my struggles but I could never stick to anything. I even had bought a stair-climbing machine after my daughter was born but it killed me to do even five minutes on the thing. I would get off of it huffing and puffing with my legs screaming so I gave that up after a couple of disappointing weeks. I'm surprised I lasted even that long!

I had pretty much decided that I was just one of those people that was not going to be an "exerciser". I could live with that. I was going to accept reality and stop feeling guilty or that I was less than anyone else because I couldn't run and didn't even want to.

Over the years while I was figuring out all of my non-diet ideas, I was taking my own advice and looking around at other people so that I could realize that no one was perfect. I ended up noticing something else in the bargain.

Everyone I observed who exercised looked so much younger than they really were and so much healthier than everyone else.

What was up with that? My then-husband has an aunt who is about 10 years older than me. All she does is walk. No big huge, leg-screaming effort. She walks for about 45 minutes just about every day. WOW! You wouldn't believe how good she looks. She could easily pass for at least 10 years younger than she really is and she is in great shape.

Then there was my next-door neighbor. She was never what I would call fat, but she was sort of pudgy. She was *soft* looking, if you know what I mean. Well, we didn't talk that much but one day I got a glimpse of her walking into her house in a spandex cat suit. *What the heck was going on here?* I asked myself. The next-door neighbor I had last seen should not be wearing a cat suit but this one was and she was looking mighty fine! *Hmmm.*

So I told her that she looked wonderful and what the heck had she been doing? Was she on a diet? She told me that no, there was no diet. She had been going to the gym and taking step aerobics classes. "You're kidding?" I asked incredulous. "You sure you are not starving yourself?"

"Nope," she told me. "Just step aerobics." Well, I'll be. That was something.

Finally after a year or two of observing these amazing things and others like them, a light went on in my thick head. Maybe I could change my body if I exercised? Maybe if I started now, I could look 10 years younger 10 years from now? What did I have to lose? Maybe this step thing would work for me as well as it had for my neighbor.

I had tried in the past to run. Couldn't make it around the block without my insides feeling as if they were on fire. I had tried the aforementioned stair-climbing thing. Too hard.

Couldn't breathe and couldn't walk too well afterwards. I had tried aerobics classes for a while when I had lived in Denver but it was too hard for me to drag myself to the gym and keep going. Plus, back then I wanted to look perfect overnight so after three months, I had given up.

So I got myself out there and bought a Jane Fonda step and video. Let me tell you, I was so proud of myself the first time I finished that tape. I had kept the step on the lowest level and was so surprised that I had actually finished the whole thing on the first attempt. Maybe I had finally found something that I could stick to!

I ended up stepping every day. I loved it. It was perfect for me because I felt like I was dancing. I was so busy concentrating intensely on the steps that I forgot that I was actually working out. Plus, I had the benefit of company while I was working out (Jane Fonda and friends) but no one could see me so I didn't have to be embarrassed when I screwed up.

I bought more tapes. I gradually raised my step to the highest level. I was kicking some butt - let me tell you. After watching and working out for six months with the likes of Jane Fonda, Gin Miller (Reebok), Keli Roberts and Karen

Voight to mention a few, I was inspired to become an aerobics instructor myself.

I thought *I could do that. I have rhythm. I would love to help people get in shape and have fun doing it.* So I dialed up my local gym and found out who I had to call to become an aerobics instructor. I called the number, bought the books, paid the fee, took the one-day class and wha-la! I was an aerobics instructor.

As it turns out, aerobics instructors were in high demand (and still are) so I was able to get a job right away. Now I've been teaching for six years and still love it. In fact I'm spoiled since I love getting paid to do something that other people have to pay for!

You are probably hoping that I will tell you that I was looking wonderful in no time at all. The truth is I was pretty out of shape. Yes, I was looking better all the time, but it took months to begin to show and years for me to get completely into shape. It truly depends on how far one has to go. If you have exercised in the past but are just getting a bit "soft" then it will not take long. I, however, had pretty much not exercised since I used to ride my bike in high school.

*It's OK to Eat
Be Fit, Healthy, and NOT on a Diet*

My metabolism didn't take as long to change, however. I noticed within months that I seemed to be eating more (working out makes you hungry) but not getting any bigger. Notice that I did not say *gaining weight*. I had taken my own good advice and thrown the damned scale in the trash.

The important part is that I felt good almost right away. I had more energy and less stress. Exercise also helped me with my desire to not worry every time I ate. I knew I was working it off and that helped quite a bit with the guilt feelings that were still attacking me from time to time.

My theories

Here is where you may want to run to the hills and forget everything thing that I have said. Don't do it!

I am not going to preach to you about how you have to exercise to be successful. I am not going to tell you to do anything at all. As you just read in my story, I didn't ever want to exercise.

Ever.

No one more than I hated seeing all of those perky fitness experts on TV selling this machine or that ab thing. I hated the ads for the gyms and the equipment. They just made me feel guilty yet again because here was something else that made me less than everyone else. But something happened to make me change my mind. I personally think that it was the natural progression of things. Once I started to appreciate myself and to be good to myself, finally having the drive to get physically fit came about sort of by itself.

I know better than anyone else that someone nagging you to do something will make it the last thing that you will ever do. Don't exercise unless you have a genuine desire to do so. It will be a waste of your time otherwise. As a matter of fact, forcing yourself to do some sort of exercise that you hate or are not interested in will definitely do more harm than good.

Work on the guilt with the food and enjoying your food and being kind to yourself first. When you feel strong, when you are ready to give it a go, then here are my recommendations on exercise and keeping with it.

*It's OK to Eat
Be Fit, Healthy, and NOT on a Diet*

1) *Don't try to do too much all at once.*

Very similar to the food advice you say? It is. The same theory applies. If you try to take on too much of a change, you will get discouraged and give up. If you tell yourself that any little bit that you do is a victory, then you will make it. If you only walk, or move in any way at all for even five minutes, it will be five minutes more than you were doing. That would be a positive thing, would it not?

Here is a sample of the too-much-at-once thinking:

I wake up starting a new day. I have promised myself that I am going to start an exercise program this very day. I am going to work out on my treadmill (which cost me about 500 bucks) for an hour. After all, I have a long way to go. I don't have time to fool around.

I have to eat my breakfast first. Getting psyched up all the while, I finish my coffee and cereal and get my workout gear on. Brand new sneakers on (to go with the treadmill), I get going.

Well, my first day I make it. I'm having difficulty breathing because I pushed myself to jog on the stupid treadmill even though I wasn't ready for jogging. Like I said, I don't have time to fool around.

It was a horrible experience. I hated it.

I congratulate myself all day because I got my working out all done. (This being the only correct thing I have done so far). I can't wait until tomorrow to do it again. Well, in truth I can't wait until I have it over with tomorrow so I can spend the rest of the day congratulating myself.

The next day, I get up ready to go again. I eat my breakfast a bit more slowly this time. I get my workout in again.

I'm thinking that hell must be full of these machines.

You get the picture. Maybe I last another day, maybe more but you can just bet that exercise does not become a way of life for me. How could it? I have made it a torturous experience. Why would anyone in their right mind want to abuse themselves in this way?

It's OK to Eat
Be Fit, Healthy, and NOT on a Diet

How about if I tried it another way? What if I went a bit easier on myself?

Yes, of course you have to sweat a bit and you have to get your heart rate up there for a while but ***you do NOT have to kill yourself.*** This is not only going to make it harder for you to keep with the program, it is unhealthy! Obviously, I don't believe in that old "go for the burn" theory.

When you begin some sort of exercise routine, you should start small. Tell yourself that you are going to get moving, but that you can stop anytime. Yes, you want to get in shape but any time spent working out that you hadn't been doing previously is a bonus!

I had some days that I actually told myself that I only had to do five minutes. If I felt okay after the five minutes was over, I would try another five. *I have worked out for 45 minutes or more by only committing to five minutes at a time.*

Again, let me remind you here to never lie to yourself. If you have a down day where you get going for your five or 10 minutes and you just don't have it in you - those 10 minutes seemed like a hundred - then by all means, stop! When you stop, you make darned sure that you still congratulate yourself on the fact that you did anything at all.

Any and all movement is a victory.

2) Find something that you enjoy doing.

Now that you have realized that you have to pace yourself let's talk about the type of exercise that a person should do. The simple answer to this question is that **any type of exercise will do just fine.** The most important issue here is that you find something that you enjoy.

For me it was step aerobics and then figure skating. For my ex's aunt it is walking. For others, it is working out on machines while they watch TV (although I myself can't stand to work out on machines. All I do is stare at the timer and count the minutes). Dancing is great exercise. There is hiking, jogging, whatever. **Just MOVE**. What you need to understand is that if you don't enjoy it at all, you won't keep doing it. Believe me, there *is* something that you will like to do. Keep looking until you find it.

What you will not find out there is this: Contrary to all of the commercials selling this machine or that workout tape, you will not find something that will make you healthy and in shape without actually doing anything. In my opinion, there is no particular machine or type of exercise that will make you burn more fat with less work. **It is not the form of exercise that makes you healthy - it is exercise itself.**

3) Try to do weight bearing exercise as well as cardio-vascular.

Don't panic. I am not suggesting that all of these changes should be made all at once. In fact, I don't even recommend it. When you are ready for more, your body will tell you.

I just wouldn't be doing my job as a fitness instructor if I didn't mention that you should build your muscles as well as move them to burn fat. For one thing, as you get older your muscle mass decreases and so you need to lift a bit of weight in order to counteract the atrophy of those muscles.

When you do cardio, you are strengthening your heart, your lungs and yes, burning fat. When you lift weights you are strengthening and actually enlarging your muscles, which will result in toning your body as well as making you strong.

Strength builds confidence. Confidence makes you even stronger.

Here is a wonderful reason to do a bit of weight lifting. Your muscles are like car engines. They are the part of your body that uses up the fat. If a car has a bigger engine, it will guzzle more fuel, will it not? Well the same thing applies to your muscles. The bigger the muscles, the more fuel will be burned. Cool, huh?

In other words, when you do your cardio you are burning extra fuel while you are working out. When you build your muscle mass, you are building your fuel-burning engine so that you burn more fuel whether you are working out or not. Yes, you will burn more fat even when you are walking around the mall! Halleluiah!

Now don't go thinking that you can just lift a few weights and skip the cardio. Won't work. If you don't believe me step into a gym and check out the big guys lifting weights with the massive shoulder and chest muscles and the POTBELLIES to go with them!

On the other hand, remember if it turns out that for you weight lifting is fun and you hate the cardio part, do the weight lifting. Eventually you may feel like walking or getting onto some sort of machine as well. If it's a choice between weight lifting and nothing, then weights it is!

Annette Mucci-Haggerty

7

Small Changes - Big rewards Over Time

My Story

After my first child, my daughter, was born I began to do some soul searching into my childhood and why I turned out the way I did. I started to read a lot of books about inner children, childhood wounds, spirituality, etc. I wanted to know how I got fat in the first place. Why was I so lonely all of the time, even when I had a husband? Why did I always feel like something was missing?

I was like an investigator - reading, bouncing ideas off my friends (driving them crazy, most likely), constantly searching for answers. I knew that I had control issues. I knew that I had insecurity issues. One of my issues is my "Invisible" problem. I have always felt invisible for as long as I can remember, especially during the teen years. I actually used to go hide when I was hanging around with my friends and wait to see if anyone missed me. How sad.

When I had gotten pregnant, I was at about 115 pounds. This was good, but still I was constantly consumed with what I was eating or not eating. I still worried about gaining weight back and was still fluctuating 5 or so pounds either way. After my daughter was born I had to lose about 40 pounds. I joined a popular diet center and that got me most of the way but it was very hard to stick to. I went to bed hungry all of the time and I knew that I couldn't live that way for long.

Two and a half years later, after continuing my inner search I gave birth to my son. Again I had gained quite a bit of weight and I had started out 5-10 pounds heavier than I had with my daughter. This was when a big surge in change, a change that had been progressing bit by bit over the years, began to really take shape.

I tried the diet center for a while again, but gave up. I just couldn't do it.

Then the real, permanent change began. First of all, I decided that I was spending all of my time taking care of other people - my two kids and my husband, who was at that time not much help. It just made sense to me that if I was going to spend all of my time taking care of their needs then I was certainly not going to deprive myself of food when I wanted it.

Something inside me said, Damn it! I am tired and hungry and no one is going to take care of my needs except for ME! From now on I'm eating whatever I want whenever I want and I refuse to feel bad about it. I am working hard here and I deserve a break! (Well, something along those lines).

That is just what I did. Yes, I did pig out a bit at first but do you know what else happened? I stopped wanting to eat as much. By telling myself that I could eat whenever I wanted I eliminated that rush to eat everything NOW because tomorrow I was going to go back on the diet.

And so all of my theories on NOT dieting began to take shape.

My Theories

Here are some small changes that you can make every day that will turn into big changes over time. Remember, even a marathon runner has to run the distance one step at a time.

1) Park as far away from the mall as you can.

Stop wasting time driving around to find the nearest spot. Park in the first spot you see - preferably the farthest one away - and walk. Unless it is freezing cold or raining, this is an easy one to do.

At the gym I get the biggest kick out of the people who drive around looking for the nearest parking space to the door. Hello! They are going into the gym to *work out* for Pete's sake! Along those same lines, I couldn't believe it when I went to Las Vegas and saw the enormous groups of people milling around on those moving sidewalks. Give me a break! If you want to go gamble, get those legs in gear and MOVE!

2) Take the stairs.

This same idea can apply anytime you are in a place that has escalators and elevators. Stairs work the biggest muscles in your body, therefore burning lots of fat.

Think of how many flights of stairs you can add to your life in just six months!

3) *Eat Popsicles.*

Popsicles are a wonderful way to do two things.

1- they help you to trick yourself into thinking that you are really eating something when you are really eating very little. After all, you have to take bites and chew, don't you? Popsicles don't have that many calories but because they are sweet, they can totally give you that feeling of satisfaction that you might need when you are not yet hungry. I used to go thru boxes of 'em!

2- they help to hold you off for a while until you get REALLY hungry.

4) *Drink lots of beverages - water in particular.*

I have found out, once I started listening to my body, that there were plenty of times that I thought I was hungry when actually I was thirsty. I was so used

It's OK to Eat
Be Fit, Healthy, and NOT on a Diet

to reaching for food that it never occurred to me that a nice big glass of Gatorade was just what I needed. Also having a sweet drink, instead of eating a cupcake would be another way to help with the sugar cravings. Try to drink plenty of fluids. You might try getting in the habit of drinking something first every time you think that you are ready to eat. This can't hurt and you'll never be dehydrated!

5) Fruit

You already know this one. Fruit is a great way to satisfy your craving for sweets and feel good about it at the same time. All natural sugar, fiber, vitamins - need I say more?

6) Go easy on the booze

Some diet "people" will tell you not to drink alcohol because of the calories. Or they will tell you to stick with the light stuff - beer and white wine. My personal feeling is that it doesn't matter what you decide to drink - just try not to do it too often or to drink too much when you do. My reasons have nothing much to do with caloric intake.

One reason is that alcohol is a depressant. It will slow your metabolism. If your metabolism slows so will your fat burning potential. Also, depressant is the opposite of what you need to keep feeling good about yourself. My advice is to proceed with caution. If you drink here and there, it shouldn't be that much of a problem.

However, there is another sneaky little glitch when you drink. I'm talking about your thinking. Everyone knows that your thinking changes when you get buzzed. It will be very hard for you to remember anything else that I've written here when you are buzzed. If there is food in front of you, you will probably just go at it with no thought as to whether you are really hungry or not. Of course, you never want to drink on an empty stomach, but you don't want to find yourself just stuffing without thinking either.

As with anything else I've said in this book, it is not my intention to tell you what to do - just what I know will help. Drinking less will help.

7) *Do something nice for someone else.*

You are probably saying to yourself, *"That's nice, but what does that have to do with the price of beans?"*

It is this. When you do something for someone else a small miracle occurs.

You stop focusing on yourself for a while. Imagine that?

One of the things that can contribute to us eating even though we are not hungry is the constant focus on ourselves. We use all of the available space in our minds thinking about how bad or empty we feel and so we focus on food to fill the void and make us feel better.

What if we did something nice for someone else instead?

We could accomplish two important things. One is that we would fill our minds temporarily with thoughts of someone else for a while and the other is that we would end up feeling awfully good.

If you don't believe me then try it. Do something nice for someone for no reason. Maybe there is someone who is going through a bad time or just someone who you think could benefit from a bit of nice attention. The trick to this is to do it completely unselfishly. In other words, don't expect anything in return. It could be anything from buying someone a cup of coffee to giving someone a nice compliment to knitting a sweater. Who knows?

The end result is that you will end up feeling really good about yourself and that will go a long way towards filling that hole inside of you instead of stuffing it with food.

Which brings me to my next suggestion.

8) Pamper yourself

Take yourself out for a manicure, pedicure, facial, or a massage. Doing nice things for yourself will help you to want to do nice things for other people. If you are going to believe that you are special then you have to put your actions to the test.

You can't say to yourself, "I'm special" and then spend all of your time cooking, cleaning, working, taking care of other people in your life and never taking care of yourself. Putting your own well being first is true self-love and makes you all the more capable of taking care of the loved ones in your life.

Also, doing nice things for yourself will help you when the time comes for you to forgive yourself for some indiscretion that you may feel that you have committed (food wise). As a matter of fact, that is the best time to do something nice for yourself - when you think you deserve it the least. That is what unconditional love is all about - not having to earn kindness. How are you going to give it to someone else (your kids, for example) if you can't give it to yourself?

Don't think I don't know how difficult it can be to do this. When you are in the habit of beating yourself up, it takes a quite a bit of practice to start doing the opposite. If you keep with it, eventually it will become second nature.

9) *Keep busy.*

Sitting still and meditating is always a good thing but when you're craving food and you are not actually hungry keeping those hands busy can help quite a bit.

I love to knit or crochet while I watch TV. It's very hard to get anything done if I have to stop every two minutes to take a bite of something. Reading a book is good also. It's very difficult to turn pages and hold onto the book if you are holding onto a bag of chips. Plus you get grease all over the pages. That stinks.

10) Start doing some investigation into what prompts you to feel so bad about yourself in the first place.

For me, reading saved my life. I began with Dr. Harville Hendrix's "Keeping the Love You Find". Then I moved onto "The Road Less Traveled" by M. Scott Peck. My all time favorite is Deepak Chopra, "Quantum Healing."

The point here is to look inward - not to feel sorry for yourself, but to do some honest soul searching. This will go a long way towards inner peace, which leads to needing to eat, shop, drink, beat ourselves and others up, etc. a lot less.

11) Share

Sometimes I will buy myself something that I seem to be craving terribly but it's just too big to eat all alone. Unfortunately, this something is not something that would taste good later, or something I even want to have around later. (pizza, muffin, bagel, bag of aforementioned chips, etc.)

What I do to remedy this situation is to offer half to anyone who is in my immediate area. I do this before I start eating so that I won't be tempted to talk myself into eating the whole thing. This is a great way to be nice to someone else and yourself at the same time.

12) Take pride in your appearance

Looking your best always makes you feel better about yourself. If you are feeling good, you are less apt to reach for something that you don't need in order to abuse yourself.

When you are feeling crappy, you usually will look crappy. Who feels like taking a shower, putting effort into accessories, doing his/her hair when she feels like cow-pucky? What I'm saying to you is that if you make an effort to look your best you will feel better inside. If you feel better inside, you will look better on the outside. Do you see a pattern here?

The same thing goes with a smile. I have personally tried to paste a smile on my face even when I don't feel like it. Sure enough, if I keep it up my smile will sink in and become genuine. Maybe it's because the people around me responded to me better if I had a smile on my face instead of a puss.

You think?

8

Perception - an extremely powerful thing.

It wasn't until I had thought that this book was complete and I was searching for some old pictures of myself from when I was "heavy" that I realized I had left this important issue out. Perception.

Here's what happened: as it turns out, there are very few fat pictures of me simply because I hated looking at pictures of myself. I also hated (and still do) posing for pictures. I was asking friends and family to see if they had any chubby pictures of me to post on my website so I could show everyone how different I look now that I've decided that I like myself and gotten rid of the "diet mentality".

My oldest friend, Jane, came over with a couple of pictures from my high-school years. "Good," I said. "You found them!"

"Well," she answered me in an apprehensive tone, "I found some pictures... but honestly, Annette, you don't look that fat to me."

What could she be talking about? Of course I was a fat teenager! Look how miserable I was over it! She was probably just trying to make me feel good, right?

WELL... I looked at the pictures, bracing myself to see that poor chubby young woman.

Strange. That chubby, unhappy young woman that I remembered myself to be was really not very chubby at all. No, I was not *skinny. But certainly, I was not what I would call FAT.*

What does this tell you? What it tells me is that my perspective was all screwed up! I PERCIEVED myself to be overweight - probably because I didn't look like a fashion model (I believe Twiggy was all the rage as I was growing up) and so all of my teen-age experiences were based on that perception.

I wonder how much happier I could have been if I had chosen to see myself differently?

Maybe, if I weren't embarrassed to change into shorts in the school locker room, or even be *seen* in shorts, I would have played sports. That surely would have kept me in good shape, don't you think?

What a shame that I wasted my teenage years beating myself up over looking bad, feeling bad about myself and denying myself a lot of the fun that I should have had -because of my negative self perception!

I will promise you this: I will not let my daughter make the same mistake. I tell her every day that she is beautiful and special. I will NEVER give her grief over how much food she eats or how she looks. I always tell her, "If you are hungry, EAT!" Food and fat will not be an issue is her life. Not if I can help it.

Now here is another story about perception that I recently remembered.

Back when I was in my early twenties, I used to hang around at my friend's boutique. As a result, I was always looking at the clothes and putting everything on layaway that I could. My paycheck usually went mostly to my friend, Judy!

I was about a size 5-ish at the time.

One day, I was admiring a particular pair of jeans. They were a size 4. I was holding them up to myself and thinking how much I liked them and how it was a damn shame that I was too fat to fit into them. (Even at a size 5, I was feeling fat. Can you believe it?)

Anyway, a cute girl came in and tried them on. She was very thin, I thought, and in great shape. Those jeans looked marvelous on her. I was envious of her that she could wear them. Funny thing though, she decided that she didn't like them and didn't buy them after all.

Hmmmm.

After she left Judy said, "Why don't you try them on if you like them? They will fit you!"

"No way will those little jeans fit me!" I said. "I'm not as thin as that girl was! I'll be lucky if I can get one leg in them."

Judy would not give up so I went in the fitting room just to shut her up.

Guess what?

The jeans fit. Not only did they fit, they looked pretty good on me. I bought them.

What this tells me and should tell you is that our perception of our size and our selves truly shapes how we go through life.

I felt fat and unattractive as a teenager and as a result, I ended up getting bigger and bigger. Yes, I did finally lose the weight, but did I even then feel good about myself? NO!!

It wasn't until I taught myself that I was indeed special and beautiful that I allowed myself to become just that.

Annette Mucci-Haggerty

9

You're On Your Own Now
(You CAN Do It)

My Story

Here is my own small story of triumph that I thought would be a great way to illustrate to you how far I have come from that miserable young woman that you met in the introduction.

I've already told you that I started doing step aerobics in my living room right after my son was born. About six months into that time, I was watching the winter Olympics and admiring the figure skating as I always did. It had been a dream of mine since I was a little girl, skating on the pond down the street from my house, to be a figure skater. I used to go down there alone in the mornings so that no one could interrupt my fantasies of skating around the pond to beautiful

It's OK to Eat
Be Fit, Healthy, and NOT on a Diet

music (playing only in my head), performing daring acts of skill on the ice. In actuality, I had never even managed to get the hang of stopping and used to just glide into a friend or just sit down on the ice to get myself stopped.

As I've said, I watched the entire Olympics thinking about how I had always wanted to be able to turn on one foot (which I now know is called a "three point turn") and maybe even do some sort of jump. As I watched, that wonderful new voice that I had cultivated inside of my head - the one that shuts up that *other* voice began to ask me, "Why can't you? Why don't you go take some lessons and learn to do those things?"

WOW! What a thought! Why, indeed shouldn't I go learn to do those things? So what if I was 32 years old? There must be someone who would teach a grown up how to skate. I called up my local skating rink and found out that the group there did in fact have a beginner program for adults.

I will never forget how much fun I had at my first lesson and how wonderful it felt to walk out of that rink knowing how to do a snow-plow stop! No more sitting down on the ice for me!

Annette Mucci-Haggerty

Over the next months I hired a skating coach. Her name was Diane Johnson and she was actually third in the Nationals Pair Competition in 1964. Luckily for me I had a pro for a teacher. She was wonderful. In six months of skating about five times a week (I used to beg my mother to watch my son and daughter for an hour while I went to the rink) I was doing my three-point turns and could even do a waltz-jump. Imagine me - someone who had given up on ever being athletic at all - figure skating and doing jumps! My jumps were nothing spectacular mind you but both of off my feet left the ice at the same time. Hey, that was good enough for me!

It turned out that there were a few other adults who were taking lessons. I found out that the skating clubs even have a category at competitions where we could skate against other adults who had not started skating as children. With the help of my coach I entered the next competition sponsored by my club. She taught me a one and one-half-minute minute program and I practiced like I was going to the Olympics.

This was a huge thing for me. I was only competing against one other woman but this other woman was few years younger than me (at least five) and had been skating for two years, where I had only been at it for six months. I found out quite a lot about myself during that time. In fact, that was when I came up with the "forgive myself" theory.

Here's how. Whenever I made a mistake in my program, that evil voice inside of me would say, *"That's it! You blew it. Just give up. It's no good now."* During my lessons, the brilliant Diane would tell me, "You can't quit like that. Even if you make a mistake, you have to keep going. If you get into the habit of stopping every time that you goof up, you will do it on the day of the competition."

Needless to say, she was right. I still struggled until I realized that I had to learn to forgive myself. Just like God would do. Just like I would do for my own children. If I make a mistake, I have to let it go and just keep going.

On the day of the competition, I was nervous as anyone could be. Before going out onto the ice I went over to my coach and she gave me the best, longest hug that I had ever gotten in my life - another moment I will never forget (thank you, Diane). I went out onto the ice and waited for my music to start, at that point pretty much in control of myself. Once the music started I fell apart. I let that stupid voice in for just a second and it was as if someone had hit me in the stomach with a brick. I couldn't even breathe correctly.

I performed the first third of my program abominably. Then something wonderful happened. I let go. I thought to myself, *Well, I can't just walk off of the ice and leave. I might as well just get this over with as best as I can.* Wouldn't you know it - the rest of the routine went off perfectly?

Luckily for me, my coach had the foresight to repeat all of my elements over again in case I screwed them up the first time. As long as you perform them correctly once you are okay.

I was very okay. I won the gold medal.

"You were only competing against one other person," you say. I don't care. I was on top of the world.

You see it wasn't the other person that I had won against. My only competition out there was myself and finally I had let myself win.

Now that I am an aerobics instructor, people are always coming up to me to ask me advice about losing weight and exercise.

It's OK to Eat
Be Fit, Healthy, and NOT on a Diet

"I'm only eating 2000 calories a day and I work my abs constantly but I can't get rid of this stomach," they say. Or, "My thighs just won't get smaller. I work out all of the time," (and those women sure do. I see them in there working like the devil himself was pushing them). "But they just stay so HUGE."

I look at them and most of the time I say, "Are you kidding? You look wonderful! What are you trying to do, kill yourself?"

Then they will usually tell me, "I can't believe that you were ever as big as you say that you were. Look at you. You are tiny. How did you do it?"

"Oh yes, I was quite the chub," I tell them. "How did I do it? I started appreciating myself for what I am and stopped dieting."

They look at me as if I have two heads. "Get out!" they say finally.

"Yup, you heard me right. I stopped dieting. I do not count calories, fat grams or weigh myself. Ever."

Unfortunately they never really believe me and I usually don't have time to go into detail. So that is what I have done right here.

You have to believe that you, like me, can have a new life. Turn everything around and do it differently. This new life does not begin, as you have probably thought in the past when you lose "X" amount of poundage or fit into whatever outfit you have hanging in your closet. This new life begins the moment you have that tiny *shift* in your way of thinking - that little *click* when you allow yourself to realize that you deserve a break and decide to give yourself that break.

You are already awesome and capable of anything. I don't care how much you weigh or what you look like. Choose to believe that and keep telling yourself that until it sinks in and I promise you, everything will change.

I want to remind you that I am only an aerobics instructor and not a doctor. I am not telling you to go ahead and eat tubs of fat if your doctor has put you on some kind of diet. What I'm hoping is that you can learn something from my mistakes and my triumphs. I am hoping that maybe you can apply one or as many of my ideas as you want to your own life and the way that you think about food. Maybe you can just get the idea that you are not alone in your struggle and that this food problem can be overcome. If this benefits you at all, then I've done what I've set out to do.

If however, you should find that you want to accept all of my ideas totally and try them for yourself then understand that you will need to decide that you have FAITH in your body, yourself, and your higher power to stick with this. What may happen (will probably happen) when you let all of your RULES about eating go is that you may pig out for a few days. I know I did. This is when it will be the hardest for you to STAND FIRM and NOT do all of the things to yourself that you are used to doing. Do NOT allow that nasty voice to come to the top of your mind. Do NOT panic and try to make up for your eating the next day. This will be the time that you have to re-read everything that I have written, write your new script for the new tape to play in your head. If you stick with it, everything will settle down and you will find that the pigging out gets boring.

On the other hand, it could turn out that you are not ready yet or in the correct frame of mind for change right now. What I've done here is to plant a seed. It may be immediate or it may be years from now that it will begin to grow. Just keep your eyes and your mind open and you will be fine.

At the very least, give yourself some sort of break. Learn that you don't have to keep beating yourself up. Learn that you can become the special person that you already have it in you to be. I like to think of Dorothy in the Wizard of OZ, when the good witch tells her that she always had the power to go home - she just didn't know it. Well, you have been born with the power. Maybe no one told you that you had it. Well, I'm telling you now that you DO! How do I know? I've been where you are and you and I are not so very different.

I wish you the best of luck. You deserve it!

It's OK to Eat
Be Fit, Healthy, and NOT on a Diet

If you have any ideas or comments that you would like to share please visit my website: Itsoktoeat.com

Hope to hear from you!

Annette Mucci-Haggerty

Annette Mucci-Haggerty

About the Author

Annette Mucci-Haggerty is an AFAA certified aerobics instructor in Massachusetts. She is also the proud mother of two beautiful children who thoroughly enjoys helping people to feel good about themselves.

CPSIA information can be obtained at www.ICGtesting.com
Printed in the USA
LVOW111911240412

278961LV00001B/63/A